Generis

PUBLISHING

Transcriptomics:New Approach to Study Genetic Alteration in T2DM

Dr. Talib Yusuf Abbas Hussain
Dr. S.H.Talib

Title: *Transcriptomics: New Approach to Study Genetic Alteration in T2DM*

Author: *Dr. Talib Yusuf Abbas Hussain, Dr. S.H.Talib,*

ISBN: 978-1-63902-501-5

Cover image: www.pixabay.com

Publisher: Generis Publishing
Online orders: www.generis-publishing.com
Contact email: info@generis-publishing.com

ABOUT THE AUTHORS

Dr. Talib Yusuf Abbas Hussain – B.Sc (Microbiology, Chemistry and Zollogy), Masters in Bioinformatics, completed his Ph.D in Medical Biotechnology.

Currently serving as a Dean (Academic Affairs), Burhani College,10-Nesbit Road, Mazgaon, Mumbai. He is also associated with MGM University, Aurangabad as a visiting faculty in the field of Bioinformatics and Biotechnology, He is popular among under graduate, Graduate and post graduate student as Examiner, Setter and Moderator.

Talib Yusuf has uptil now published more than 35 Research articles in international and national peer reviewed journal with good impact factor.

Previously Talib Yusuf has served as Asst Professor and Head of the dept, Dept of Biotechnology, Dr. Rafiq Zakaria Campus, Maulana Azad College, Rauza Bagh, Aurangabad, having teaching experience of 15 Years.

Dr. S.H.Talib - Dr. S.H. Talib, MD (Medicine), MD (Chest), Ph.D, FICA, FCCP, Prof Emeritus, Internal Medicine, Govt Medical College & Hospital, Aurangabad-431001, India.
Former Prof. & Head, Professor Emeritus, Dept. of Medicine, MGM Medical College & Hospital, Aurangabad-431001, India.

S. H. Talib served as senior professor and head at the Department of Medicine Mahatma Gandhi Mission's medical college, Aurangabad, Maharashtra India. He also has had over three decades association with Government Medical College, Aurangabad from where he retired as chief of Department of Medicine and then joined the prestigious Mahatma Gandhi Mission's Medical College as professor and head in 2006 and retired in 2018. Presently continuing as Professor Emeritus and Chief Advisor to Department of Medicine.

Dr. Talib also served as chairman of board of studies in medicine, senior member of academic council and was a member at management council of MGM institute of Health Sciences, Navi Mumbai. He served as advisor to Drug Controller General of India, Nirman Bhavan, New Delhi; several committees of Government medical education and drug department, Maharashtra State, India.

He is an experienced clinical teacher, responsible for teaching and training undergraduate and post graduate students of different specialties. He is recipient of several prestigious awards and honors including Professor Emeritus in Medicine at Government Medical college, Aurangabad, MGM medical college, Aurangabad and lifetime achievement awards. A teacher par excellence, and was a very popular examiner for Under-graduate and Post-graduate students of medicine of several universities all over India. He is a pioneer member in establishing the allergy clinics at Aurangabad, awarded fellowships of Indian & American college of allergy, asthma and immunology. He is also a founder member of Indian society of sleep disorders, New Delhi.

He has contributed many chapters in updates of medicine and has over 110 scientific publications in National and International journals and published a book entitled "Essentials in Respiratory Medicine". He has also organized historic National and International conferences of ICAAI in 2011 and International convention on challenges in medical education (2015). He keeps special interest in diabetology as physician.

He has two more books under print, An Evidence based symptom analysis bag of tricks for learning students of medicine and Illustrative Review in Clinical Pulmonology. Nearing age of seventy three, maintains an active clinical research attitude and practice.

ACKNOWLEDGEMENTS

The completion of this book has been one of the most significant academic challenges I have ever had to face. The journey towards the completion of this book was an unforgettable learning experience. This book has been kept on track and been seen through to completion.

with the support and encouragement of numerous people including my teachers, colleagues, my friends and well-wishers. Without the guidance, support and patience of all the concerned persons, this study would be unattainable. It is to them I owe my deepest gratitude.

I am lucky in having Dr. S.N.Harke, Professor and Principal, Dept of Biotechnology, MGM School of Biomedical Sciences, Aurangabad, and Dr. S.H.Talib, Head & Professor,Department of Medicine, MGM Medical College and Hospital, Aurangabad and I am greatly indebted to them for their time to time guidance for providing the vision, encouragements and advices necessary to proceed through and carry forward the write up and analysis, and encouragements that I had gained, changed my perspective towards the research.

I sincerely thank to Dr. Rajesh Dase, PSM dept, MGM Medical College and Hospital, Aurangabad, for statistical analysis and Dr.Ashok Shinde, MGM IBT, Aurangabad, Mr.Balasaheb Warkhade, Professor, Model College, Ghansawangi, for their valuable suggestions in genomic interpretations.

I would like to thank Xcelris Lab Ltd, Ahmedabad for their kind assistance in Next Generation Sequencing and transcriptome analysis.

Lastly indebted to my Mother, Late Father, my Wife for bearing with me patiently during my completion of this herculious task. I owe important dept to my kids Farida and Taha who considered my work as a fun.

Talib Yusuf Abbas Husain

Abbreviations

ADA	American Diabetes Association
ApoB	Apolipoprotein B
BMI	Body mass index
BP	Blood pressure
CD/CV	Common disease – common variant
CEU	U.S. residents with northern and western European ancestry
CHD	Coronary heart disease
CHR	Chromosome
CNV	Copy number variation
CVD	Cardiovascular disease
DCCT	Diabetes Control and Complication Trail
DGI	Diabetes Genetics Initiative
DIAGRAM	Diabetes Genetics Replication And Meta-analysis Consortium
DNA	Deoxyribonucleic acid
EWA	Environment-wide association
FPKM	Fragments per kilobase per million reads mapped
FPG	Fasting plasma glucose
FUSION	Finland-United States Investigation of NIDDM Genetics
GAD	Glutamic acid decarboxylase
GDM	Gestational diabetes mellitus
GI	Gastrointestinal
GIANT	Genetic Investigation of Anthropometric Traits

GoKinD	Genetics of Kidneys in diabetes study
GWAS	Genome-wide association studies
GTF	Gene Transfer file
HbA1c	Glycated hemoglobin
HDL	High-density lipoprotein
HLA	Human leukocyte antigen
HOMA-IR	Homeostasis model assessment of insulin resistance
HUNT	The Nord-Trøndelag Health Survey
HUNT1	The first Nord-Trøndelag Health Survey
HUNT2	The second Nord-Trøndelag Health Survey
HWE	Hardy-Weinberg equilibrium
HISAT	Hierarchical indexing for spliced alignment of transcripts
IDF	International Diabetes Federation
IFG	Impaired fasting glycemia
IGT	Impaired glucose tolerance
IR	Insulin Resistance
IS	Insulin Secretion
KAAS	KEGG Automatic Annotation Server
LADA	Latent autoimmune diabetes of adults
LOG2FC	Log 2 transformed fold change values
LD	Linkage Disequilibrium
MAF	Minor allele frequency
MAGIC	The meta analysis of glucose and insulin traits consortium

MALDI-TOF	Matrix assisted laser desorption/ionization time of light
Mb	Megabase
MDC	Malmo Diet and Cancer Cohort
MI	Myocardial infarction
MODY	Maturity onset diabetes of the young
MPP	Malmo Preventive Project
mRNA	Messenger RNA
NCBI	National Center for Biotechnology Information
NCI-NHGRI	National Cancer Institute and National Human Genome Research Institute
OGTT	Oral Glucose Tolerance test
OR	Odds Ratio
PAR	Population attributable Risk
PCOS	Polycystic ovary syndrome
PCR	Polymerase Chain Reaction
QC	Quality control
TZD	Thiazolidinediones
UKT2D	UK Type 2 Diabetes
UTR	Untranslated Region
WHO	World Health Organization
WTCCC	Welcome Trust Case Control Consortium

Gene Name Abbreviations

ABCB11	ATP-binding cassette, sub family B (MDR/TAP), member 11

ABCC8	ATP-Binding cassette, sub family C (CFTR/MRP), member 8
ADAMTS9	ADAM metallopeptidase with thrombospondin type 1 motif, 9
ADCY5	Adenylate cyclase 5
ANK1	Ankyrin 1, erythrocytic
AP3S2	Adapter -related protein coplex 3, sigma 2 subunit
ARAP1	ArfGAP with RhoGAP domain, ankyrin repeat and pH domain
ATP11A	Atpase, class VI, type 11A
BDNF	Brain-derived neurotrophic factor
BLK	B lymphoid tryosinge kinase
BNC2	Basonuclin 2
C2CD4A	C2 Calcium- dependant domain containing 4 A
CDC123	Cell division cycle 123 homolog
CDKAL1	CDK5 regulatory subunits associated protein 1-like 1
CDKN2A	Cyclin dependant kinase inhibitor 2 A
CDKN2B	Cyclin depenedant kinase inhibitor 2 B
CDKN2BAS	CDKN2B antisense RNA 1 (non protein coding)
CEL	Carboxylester lipase
DGKB	Diacylglycerol kinase, beta 90kDa
DUSP9	Dual Specificity phosphatase 9
FN3K	Fructoasmine 3 kinase
FTO	Fat mass and obesity associated
G6PC2	Glucose-6-Phosphatase, catalytic, 2

GCK	Glucokinase (hexokinase 4)
GCKR	Glucokinase (hexokinase 4) regulator
GCS	Goosecoid protein
GRB14	Growth factor receptor-bound protein 14
HFE	Henochromatosis
HHEX	Hematopoietically expressed homeobox
HK1	Hexokinase 1
HMG20A	High mobility group 20A
HMGA2	High mobility group AT hook 2
HNF1A	HNF 1 homeobox A
HNF1B	HNF1 homeobox B
HNF4A	Hepatocyte nuclear factor 4, alpha
INS	Insulin
IRS1	Insulin resistance substrate 1
KCNJ11	Potassium inwardly rectifying channel, subfamily J, member 11
KCNQ1	Potassium voltage-gated channel, KQT-like subfamily, member 1
MADD	MAP-kinase activating death domain
MC4R	Melanocortin 4 receptor
MITF	Microphtalmia associated transcription factor
MTNR1B	Melatonin receptor 1B
NEUROD1	Nueronal differentiation 1
NOTCH2	Neurogenic locus notch homolog protein
PAX4	Paired Box 4

PKN2	Protein Kinase N2
PPARG	Peroxisome proliferator acticated receptor gamma
PRC1	Protein regulator of cytokinesis 1
PROX1	Prosperohomeobox 1
PTPRD	Protein tyrosine phosphatase, receptor type, D
RBMS1	RNA binding motif, single stranded interacting protein 1
SLC30A8	Solute carried family 30 (zinc transporter), member 8
SORCS1	Sortilin related VPS10 domain containing receptor 1
SPTA1	Spectrin aplha erythrocytic 1
SRR	Serine racemase
TCF7L2	Traanscription factor 7 like 2 (T cell Specific)
THADA	Thyroid adenoma associated
TLE4	Transductin like enhancer of split 4
TMPRSS6	Transmembrane protease, serine 6
TSPAN8	Tetraspanin 8
TUBGCP3	tubulin, gamma complex associated protein 3
VPS13C	Vacoular protein sorting 13 homolog C
VPS26A	Vacoular Protein sorting 26 homolog A
WDR72	WD Repeat domain 72
WFS1	Wolfram Syndrome 1 (wolframin)
ZFAND6	Zinx Finger, AN1-type domain 6
FA	Fatty acid
dNTP	Deoxyribonuclic acid
EIF	Eukaryotic translation initiation factor

GK	Glucokinase
GKRP	Glucokinase regulatory protein
IGF-1	Insulin like growth factor I
IGFBP3	Insulin like growth factor binding protein 3

List of Tables

List of Figures

List of Graphs

TABLE OF CONTENTS

24

Chapter I. Introduction

With the intensive growth of the amount of publicly available genomic data, a new field of computer science i.e., Bioinformatics has emerged, focusing on the use of computing systems for efficiently deriving, storing, and analyzing the character strings of genome to help to solve problems in molecular biology. The term Bioinformatics was coined by Paulien Hogeweg in 1979 for the study of informatics processes in biotic systems. The National Center for Biotechnology Information (NCBI, 2001) defines as Bioinformatics is the field of science in which biology, computer science and information technology merges into a single discipline. In this field there are three important sub discipline within: the development of new algorithms and statistics with which to assess relationships among members of large data sets,; the analysis and interpretation of various types of data including nucleotides, amino acid sequence, protein domains, protein structures,the development and implementation of tools that enable efficient access and management of different types of information.

Bioinformatics is the use of IT in the field of Biotechnology for the various macromolecular data storage, data warehousing and analyzing different complex macromolecular data for the study of central dogma.

The flood of data from biology, mainly in the form of DNA, RNA and Protein sequences, puts heavy demand on computers and computational scientists. At the same time, it demanDiabetic a transformation of basic ethos of biological sciences. Hence, Data mining techniques can be used efficiently to explore hidden pattern underlying in biological data in various human diseases Un-supervised classification, also known as clustering; which is one of the branches of Data Mining can be applied to biological data and this can result in a better era of rapid medical development and drug discovery. Diabetes mellitus is a endocrine metabolic disorder, it is unfortunate that India is considered diabetes capital of the globe. Necessitating researchers to probe and peep into genomic analysis of the disease with the aid of Bioinformatics.

In the past decade, the advent of efficient genome sequencing tools has led to enormous progress in life sciences. Among the most important innovations, microarray technology allows to quantify the expression for thousand of genes simultaneously. The characteristic of these data which makes it different from machine-learning/pattern recognition data includes, a fair amount of random noise, missing values, a dimension in the range of thousands, and a sample size in few dozens. A particular application of the micro array technology is undertaken in our study of diabetes research, where the goal is to search for gene expression at transcriptome level in Healthy, prediabetic and diabetic subjects, and there effects on Gene Ontology (molecular function, cellular component and Biological process) and metabolic pathways. The challenge for a biologist and computer scientist is to provide solution based on terms of automation, quality and efficiency in understanding genomic information in abnormal glycemic state between healthy individual and diabetes.

Pre diabetes and Diabetes:-

The global prevalence of pre diabetes has been increasing progressively in past few decades, As per IDF (international diabetes federation) diabetes Atlas, the number of cases IGT (Impaired Glucose Tolerance) To worldwide is estimated to be approximately 340 million (2). By 2030 the global prevalence of IGT is estimated to reach 8.4% which will be approximately 462 million people. It has been established that pre-diabetic status is a strong risk factor for overt diabetes with or without Micro and Macro vascular complications. (1,2).

Type 2 Diabetes is a complex disease that is caused by a complex interplay between genetic, epigenetic and environmental factor Diabetes refers to a group of metabolic diseases characterized by hyperglycemia resulting from defects in insulin secretion, insulin action, or both. (3). The chronic hyperglycemia of diabetes is associated with long term damage, dysfunction, and failure of different organs, like eye, kidneys, nerve, heart and blood vessels. Diabetes is currently fastest growing epidemic and has been ascribed to a collision between genes and the environment.

Normal glucose tolerance is maintained by following Mechanism-

a)   Insulin secretion occurs from pancreas in response to carbohydrate load.
b)   Suppression of endogenous hypatic glucose production of insulin.'
c)   Insulin mediated glucose uptake by peripheral insulin responsive tissue like muscle and fat.

In Type 2 Diabetes glucose uptake by peripheral tissue is decreased due to development of resistance to insulin. These resistance occurs 5 to 10 Years or even more before development of Diabetes Mellitus. These period is considered prediabetic where pancreas working overtime when patient develop full blown diabetes the pancreas is still working overtime and get exhausted. This is considered so called Clinical Diabetes

Mellitus. The pancreas tries to overcome this resistance initially by producing more insulin leading to hyperinsulinaemic state. When the overproduction of insulin by pancreas fail to overcome the insulin resistance, clinical diabetes, develops late insulin secretion starts declining either due to glucose toxicity and B-cell exhaustion. Increase in hepatic glucose production also seen in Type 2 Diabetes (T2D) but not in Impaired Glucose Tolerance (IGT). These increased hepatic glucose production is reversible with lifestyle modification and oral agents.

T2D have a strong genetic component although identification of susceptibility genes have been elusive and no single gene defect explained T2D; hence the disease is heterogenic, multigenic and has complexitiology.(4).

Genome Wide Associations Studies (GWAS) :-

Genome-wide association studies (GWAS) have facilitated a substantial and rapid rise in the number of confirmed genetic susceptibility variants for type 2 diabetes (T2D). Approximately 40 variants havebeen identified so far, many of which were discovered through GWAS in available literature (11). This success has led to widespread hope that the findings will translate into improved clinical care for the increasing numbers of patients with diabetes. Potential areas or clinical translation include risk prediction and subsequent disease prevention, pharmacogenetics, and the development of novel therapeutics. However, the genetic loci so far identified account for only a small fraction (approximately 10%) of the overall heritable risk for T2D. Uncovering the missing heritability is essential to the progress of T2D genetic studies and to the translation of genetic information into clinical practice.[7].

Next Generation Sequencing (NGS) and Genome Wide Association Studies (GWAS):-

NGS (next generation sequencing) and GWAS (Genome Wide association studies) have led to technical development of genetic variants risked and protection of Type 2 Diabetes Mellitus. Next Generation Sequencing (NGS) which shows the amount of gene which has been expressed and there arrangement of nucleotide bases in the gene fragments which codes for protein, also some genes, or a copy of a gene which has lost the ability to produce a functional protein, may be due to mutation or inaccurate duplication in the sequence which can be termed as pseudogene. [11]. Pseudogene expression can be found due to Single Nucleotide Polymorphism (SNP's), are DNA variant that occur when a single base pair (A,T,G and C) in the sequence altered.

Transcriptome Analysis:-

Transcriptome analysis is an important tool for characterization and understanding of the molecular basisof phenotypic variation in biology, including diseases. During the past decades micro-arrays have been the most important and widely used approach for such analyses, but recently high-throughput sequencing of cDNA (RNA-seq) has emerged as a powerful alternative present study is based on this new transcriptome analysis (5). And it has already found numerous applications (4). RNA-seq uses next-generation sequencing (NGS) methods to sequence cDNA that has been derived from an RNA sample, and hence produces millions of short reads. These reads are then typically mapped to a reference genomeand the number of reads mapping within a genomic feature of interest (such as a gene or an exon) is usedas a measure of the abundance of the feature in the analyzed sample. Arguably the most common use of transcriptome profiling is in the search for differentially expressed genes (DEG), that is, genes that show differences in expression level between conditions or in other ways are associated with given predictors or responses. RNA-seq offers several advantages over microarrays for differential expression analysis, such as an increased dynamic range and a lower background level, and the ability to detect and quantify the expression of previously unknown transcripts and isoforms [7,8,9].

The Global prevalence of pre-diabetes and diabetes have been increasing progressively from past few decades and India being a major hub centre for Diabetes Mellitus globally of this world.

Present study is therefore undertaken pre diabetic and diabetic for recognizing genes which have been expressed and their arrangements of nucleotide base in the gene fragments which code for protein and also to recognize the genes which has lost their ability to produce functional proteins and genes. We have humbly tried to analyze with purity and concentration of Nanodrop Spectrophotometer of RNA, central dogma sstudy, gene ontology and metabolic pathway analysis for differential expressed genes in Healthy, Prediabetic and Diabetic Subjects. To best of my knowledge and search of literature finger countable studies on RNA-Seq (Transcriptome) on diabetes and prediabetic samples are available in the Indian and Western literature.

Chapter II. Aim and Objectives

Aim

Analysis and Data Mining of Gene Expression Studies using Microarray Technologies andBioinformatics in Type 2 Diabetes Mellitus (T2DM).

Objectives

Following objectives will be covered during the proposed research work:

a) To study the functions of genes involved Type 2 Diabetes Mellitus, Pre diabetic and healthy withreference genome.

b) To identify and isolate neo recognized Single Nucleotide Polymorphism (SNP's) andPseudogenes in samples of Diabetic, Prediabetic, and Healthy subjects.

c) To document and analyse Gene Ontology (GO) (Cellular components, Biological processes, Molecular functions) and any differentially expressed genes (DEG) involved in metabolic pathway, cell regulations of Diabetic, Prediabetic, and Healthy Subjects.

Chapter III. Review of Literature

3A-Bioinformatics

Bioinformatics [12], [13], [14], [15] is the application of Computer Science technology to the field of Biology specially in Molecular Studies like DNA, RNA and Protein (Amino Acids). The term Bioinformatics was coined by Paulien Hogeweg in 1978 for "*The study of informatics processes in biotic systems*". The National Centre for Biotechnology Information (NCBI, 2001) defines Bioinformatics as "the field of science in which Biology, Computer Science, and Information Technology merges into a single discipline". There are three important areas in Bioinformatics:

1) The development of new algorithms and statistics with which to assess relationships among membersof large data sets.
2) the analysis and interpretation of various types of data including nucleotide and amino acid sequences, protein domains, and protein structures.
3) And the development and implementation of tools that enable efficient access and management of different types of information.
4) The explosive growth in the amount of biological data demanDiabetic the use of computing systems for the organization, the maintenance and the analysis of biological data.

The aims of Bioinformatics are:

1) The organization of data in such a way that allows researchers to access existing information and tosubmit new entries as they are produced.
2) The development of tools that help in the analysis of data.
3) The use of these tools to analyze the individual systems in detail, in order to gain new biological insights.

In this present study our focus is to implement different methods, programs, Algorithms to study differential expressed genes and correlating with metabolic pathways focusing on Diabetes MellitusType II.

Application of Data Mining techniques to Bioinformatics

Certain sub areas in Bioinformatics where data mining can be utilized to explore explicit informationin molecular data. [12], [13]. Some of the areas are described below in brief:

Data mining in Gene Expression: Gene expression analysis can be used to study and analyze the expression based on mRNA's (the process by which a gene's coded information is converted into the structural and functional units of a cell) in order to characterize biological processes and elucidate the mechanisms of gene transcription [12].

Data mining in genomics: Genomics is the study of an organism's genome and deals with the systematic use of genome information to provide new biological knowledge [13].

Data Mining in Proteomics: Proteomics is the large-scale study of proteins. Data mining can be used particularly for prediction of protein's structures and functions [15].

Present work is focused too study and analyse Gene Ontology which highlight their molecular function, biological process and cellular components of Diabetes mellitus Type II.

Introduction to Microarray Technology:-

Compared with the traditional approach to genomic research, which is focused on the local examination and collection of data on single genes [16], microarray can simultaneously measure the expression level of thousands of genes within a particular sample. Such high throughput expression profiling canbe used to compare the level of gene transcription in clinical conditions in order to: - I) identify diagnostic or prognostic biomarkers; II) Classify diseases; III) monitor the response to therapy; and IV) understand the mechanisms involved in genesis of disease processes. [17-26]. For these reasons, DNA microarrays are considered important tools for discovery in clinical medicine.

The two major types of microarray experiments are the cDNA microarray and oligonucleotide arrays (abbreviated oligo chip). Despite differences in the details of their experiment protocols, both types of experiments involve three common basic procedures ([12], [13], [14]) :

Chip manufacture: A microarray is a small chip (made of chemically coated glass, nylon membrane or silicon), onto which tens of thousands of DNA molecules (probes) are attached in fixed grids. Each grid cell relates to a DNA sequence.

Target preparation, labeling and hybridization: Typically, two mRNA samples (a test sample and a control sample) are reverse-transcribed into cDNA (targets), [27] labeled using either fluorescent dyes or radioactive isotopic, and then hybridized with the probes on the surface of the chip.

The scanning process: Chips are scanned to read the signal intensity that is emit-ted from the labeled and hybridized targets [28].

Generally, both cDNA microarray and oligo chip experiments measure the expression level for each DNA sequence by the ratio of signal intensity between the test sample and the control sample, therefore, data sets resulting from both methods share the same biological semantics. Next Generation Sequencing (NGS), an advancement of Microarray has been utilized here.

In this thesis work NGS has been implemented by hiring services of Xcelris Lab, Ltd, Ahmedabad, for sequencing process where transcripts reads had been obtained and further statistical andGO (Gene ontology) Analysis performed.

3B -Gene Expression Data

Microarray experiment allows description of GWA (Genome Wide Association) expression change in health and disease. Microarray is a multiplex lab on a chip (figure 1). It is a 2D array on a solid substrate that assays large amount of biological material using high throughput screening methods. Microarray helps in estimating the amount of protein in the cell and a lot of information can be derived from this technology. Hence, microarrays provide a tool for answering a wide range of questions about the dynamics of cell. Microarray technology is used for two reasons:- I) to identify the sequence of gene and II) to determine the expression level of genes (figure 2).

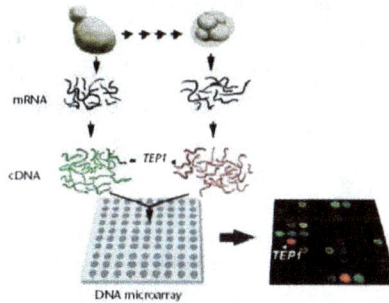

Figure 1. DNA microarray

Microarray Technology: Overview of gene expression analysis using a DNA microarray.[29]

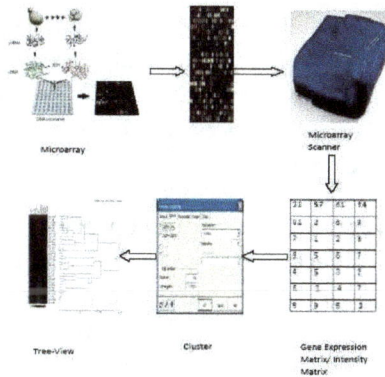

Figure 2. Gene Expression Analysis process

Complete Overview of Gene Expression Analysis, isolation from cell to analysis till tree view inevolutionary tree and their gene ontology.

Genetic mapping in Human Diseases

Genetic mapping is a powerful approach used for identification of genes underlying any trait influenced by inheritance, including human diseases. The methodology is based on the correlation between trait andDNA variation and is carried out without the need for prior hypotheses about biological function [30]. Ever since the rediscovery of Mendel's laws of inheritance in the early 1900s and the subsequent awareness that most naturally

33

occurring phenotype variation involves the action of multiple genes and non-genetic factors, geneticists have searched for practical tools for discovering genes contributing to human diseases. Human genetic variation was termed "breakthrough of the year" by Science in 2007 [31], reflecting the recent years' striking progress in understanding the genetic basis underlying normal human phenotypic variation and susceptibility to a wide range of diseases [32].

Classification of genetic variants

A gene is a unit of hereditary in a living organism. To understand a genome more comprehensively, we need to move beyond the static view and understand how genes interact with each other. Genetic information in the gene is contained in the form of DNA [31]. The basic complement of DNA in an organism is called the genome. The human genome is packed in two sets of 23 chromosomes; one set inherited from each parent whose own DNA is a mosaic of preceding ancestors. Consequently, the human genome functions as a diploid unit with phenotypes arising due to the complex interplay of alleles of genes and/or their non-coding functional regulatory elements [32]. The haploid human genome consists of approximately 3 billion nucleotides, in each cell. Among two random individuals the genomes vary by approximately 0.5% [33]. This variation affects the majority of human phenotypic differences, from eye colour and height to disease susceptibility and responses to drugs [32].

Phenotypic diversity is determined by genetic variation acting in conjugation with environmental and behavioral factors. The genetic variants are classified by two basic criteria: their frequency in the population and their composition – i.e. sequence variants or structural variants. Sequence variation varies from single nucleotide variants to 1 kilo-base (kb) insertions or deletions (indels) of DNA segments.

Structural variation is a common designation for larger insertions and deletions, as well as duplications, inversions and translocations, ranging in size from 1 kb to more than 5 mega-bases (Mb) (Figure 4). If a DNA segment is present in variable numbers compared to the reference sequence, as in duplications, deletions or insertions, it is termed a copy number variant (CNVs) [31-34].

Figure 3. Classification of genetic variants

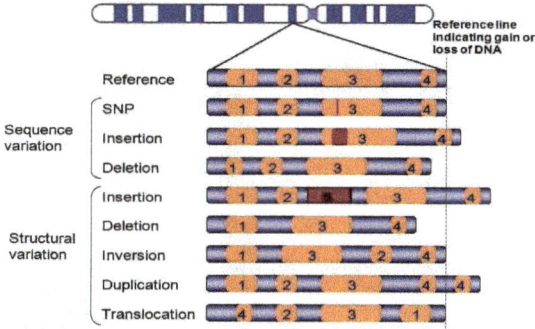

Classification of genetic variants by composition, showing examples of sequence variation and structural variation compared to a reference sequence. Modified from [31,35]

According to their frequency, genetic variants are referred to as common if their minor allele frequency (MAF) is >5% in the population, while rare variants are present at a frequency <5%. A polymorphism is, in principle, defined as a genetic variant that is present in •1% of the population. Thus, a single-nucleotide variant showing a frequency >1% is consequently termed single nucleotide polymorphism (SNP) [31]. It is estimated that the human genome harbors approximately 10 million SNPs comprising 78% of the human variants. In contrast, structural variants are estimated to account for no more than 22% of all variants, but comprise an estimated 74% of the nucleotides that may differ from person to person [33].

3C- Trasncriptomics

Mapping of genetic variants underlying human traits

Mapping of genetic variation underlying human traits depends on two key concepts: genetic linkage and linkage disequilibrium. Genetic linkage is the phenomenon where recombination between two loci occurs with less than 50% probability in a single generation; resulting in co-segregation more often than if they were independently inherited. In other words, genetic linkage is the tendency of certain alleles to be inherited together. Genetic loci that are physically close to one another on the same chromosome tend to stay together during meiosis, and are thus genetically linked [33]. The second concept, *linkage disequilibrium (LD)*, is a measure of association between alleles at separate but linked loci, usually resulting from a particular ancestral chromosomal

35

segment (haplotype) being common in the population studied. This phenomenon causes polymorphisms to be correlated to the point of being strong proxiesfor each other [36]. Different statistics have been used to measure the amount of linkage disequilibrium between two variant alleles, one of the most common being the coefficient of correlation r2 [37]. When r2 = 1, the two variant alleles are in complete linkage disequilibrium, whereas r2 < 1 indicate that the ancestral complete linkage disequilibrium has been eroded. Due to this phenomenon of LD, it is possible to choose a subset of highly informative SNPs, or "tag" SNPs, to represent certain haplotypes, and the number of SNPs to be genotyped in a larger sample can therefore be reduced without losing the ability to capture most of the variation. For example, it is possible to select a set of 300,000 to one million SNPs torepresent most of the 10 million common SNPs estimated to be present in the human genome [36]. Because the causal SNP is often not typed within a genetic association study, it is important to cross- examine SNPs that have not been genotyped directly. This can be done through imputation. Imputation methoDiabetic predict the alleles of SNPs not directly genotyped in the study (or hidden SNPs) using thecorrelation structure (LD) between the SNPs in the region. The starting point of any imputation methodis a reference data set for which the genotypes of a dense set of SNPs are provided, such as HapMap. The fundamental assumption is that the reference samples, the cases, and the controls are all sampled from the same population. Under this simplifying assumption, the three populations share the same LD structure. Thus, the structure of the LD in the reference population, in combination with the structure of the LD of the observed SNPs within the cases and the controls, may be used to impute the alleles of a hidden SNP [38]. Several different approaches have been used in the exploration of genetic factors involved in complex disease. The progress has generally been guided by technological advances in genotyping and sequencing techniques, statistical handling of data and also by collection of larger cohorts suitable for genetic studies. In general, two methods have been used for studying genetic factors involved in human diseases in the 20th century: the so-called *candidate gene approach* and the *linkage analysis approach* [39-41]. The linkage approach has proved very effective in the identification of rare variants with a high degree of penetrance, such as those responsible for extreme forms of early-onset diseases segregating as monogenic (Mendelian) disorders – including MODY, mitochondrial diabetes with deafness, neonatal diabetes and rare forms of severe childhood obesity [42-44]. However, because the risk for relatives is lower in complex diseases due to the low penetrance of polygenic risk variants, the statistical power of this method in studies of polygenic traits is limited [45]. Even for loci with considerable effects on susceptibility at the population level, the number of families needed to offer sound power to detect linkage has proven hard to obtain [46]. Very few variants with large phenotypic effect (high-impact risk alleles) appear to be present in common complex diseases, thus most linkage studies have, in retrospect, been seriously underpowered. This could also explain the inadequate findingsand the lack of replication of regions putatively linked to disease. Moreover, even when evidence of linkage is observed, the genomic region linked to the trait of interest is often very large; hence the identification of the causal gene or genetic variant often remained the main challenge.

The candidate gene approach examines specific genes with a plausible role in the disease process. For diabetes, natural candidates are genes involved in glucose homeostasis and metabolism. Theapproach is biased since it assumes that a specific gene or loci is associated with disease before testing. The genetic variants are identified through focused sequencing and further assessed by genotyping them in a large number of cases and controls. Even though this approach has contributed to the identification of numerous published associations, only a fraction of the associations have been replicated by other studies [45-46]. There are several reasons for non-replications: a) lack of statistical power in follow-up studies to detect or exclude a previously reported finding, b) false positive findings in the initial report due to incomplete or no correction for multiple testing, c) spurious associations as a consequence of population stratification or by random, d) differences in allele frequencies or LD between the genetic variants in the populations studied, e) differences in selection and phenotypic characteristics of the study participants/cases and controls or, f) unmeasured population-specific environmental exposures that may confound the association [47-49].

Thus, methods used successfully to identify the genes underlying rare Mendelian diseases generally failed in the identification of the genetic basis of common disorders such as cancer, diabetes and heart disease. This suggested that most of the genetic contribution to complex diseases arises from multiple loci with individually small effects (Figure 5). The conceptual outline for association studies to identify common genetic variants underlying common complex diseases was first reported by Risch and colleagues in 1996 [50], and is now referred to as the common disease/common variant (CD/CV) hypothesis. The major assumption behind the CD/CV hypothesis is that since the major diseases are common, so are the genetic variants that cause them. Moreover, common variants with low penetrance and modest risk are not subjected to the same negative selection as variants with strong phenotypiceffect causing Mendelian diseases. Hence, *the hypothesis states that common diseases are caused by multiple, high frequency genetic variants conferring cumulative incremental effects on disease risk* [33,51]. With

37

these assumptions as a fundament, the next challenge became clear - to survey the common genetic variation in the genomes of a large number of individuals. This would be necessary in order to reveal the intricate genetic background of common complex diseases.

Figure 4. Allelic spectrum of disease

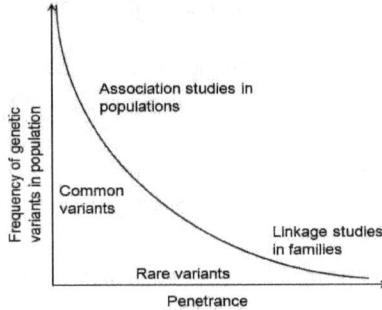

Frequency of genetic variants in population

Association studies in populations

Common variants

Linkage studies in families

Rare variants

Penetrance

The allelic spectrum of disease relies on the number of genetic variants, their frequency in a populationand on the penetrance (size of their phenotypic effect).

The allelic spectrum of disease relies on the number of genetic variants, their frequency in a population and on the penetrance (size of their phenotypic effect) [51]. Linkage studies have proved successful in identifying genetic variants causing rare Mendelian disorders, those with low-frequencyand high penetrance. Complex diseases are believed to be caused by multiple genetic variants each conferring only low to modest risk for disease [31,52].

The breakthrough came in 2006-2007 with the successful implementation of genome-wide association studies (GWAS). This new approach became possible as a result of the completion of the human genome sequence in 2001 [206, 207], the creation of SNP LD maps by the International HapMapProject [98] and great advancements in genotyping technology (efficient gene-chips) and tools for statistical handling [29]. Using SNP-based arrays and comparing the frequency of SNP alleles between cases and controls, the GWA approach allowed the investigators to detect genetic variants with modest phenotypic effects in a systematic and unbiased manner, provided that the variants had a high frequency in the population. *These studies required large numbers of patients and cost several million dollars each*. Due to the vast amount of genetic variants analyzed in a GWA study, a high number of statistical tests are performed, thus leading to a substantial risk of false positives owing to multiple testing. The important need for controlling this problem has resulted in the general use of a more stringent genome- wide significance level before an association is considered statistically significant. Current consensus has, based on a simulation study, defined a genome-wide significance level of P < 5×10-8 to account for 106 independent genome-wide hypotheses tested in a dense GWA (56), even though also P < 10-7 has been suggested (57,58).

Approximately 951 GWA studies covering over two hundred distinct diseases and traits have been published by the second quarter of 2011, with nearly 1,450 SNP–trait associations reported as significant (P <5×10í8) (Figure 4) [59,60]. The upshot is that hundreds of common genetic variants have now been statistically linked with various diseases. Such associations are consistent with the common disease–common variant hypothesis, which posits that common diseases are attributable in part to allelic variants present in more than 1–5% of the population [58-60]. Hence, genome-wide association studies have, without doubt, provided valuable insights into the genetic architecture of common complex disorders. However, most variants identified so far confer relatively small increments in risk, and explain only a small proportion of familial clustering, thus leading to question of how the remaining "missing heritability" can be explained. Possible sources of the missing heritability and future research strategies, including and extending beyond current genome-wide association approaches. SNPs play an important role in evolutionary segments which make them easier to follow the population and individual studies. SNPs do not cause disease, but they can help determine the likelihood and can correlate the dissimilarity between the classes. Of course SNPs are not absolute which indicates some relationship with disease development, someone who has inherited 2 alleles IRS4 (insulin receptor substrate), or IRS2 (insulin receptor substrate) may never develop Diabetes Mellitus Type 2, while another who has been inherited 2 alleles may develop, IRS 6 (insulin receptor substrate) is just one gene that has been linked to Diabetes Mellitus.

Apart from SNPs, pseudogene also play an important role in disease causing, because when gene loses the ability to produce protein, reason might be mutation or inaccurate duplication. Dogma has dictated that because the pseudogene no longer produces a protein it becomes functionless and evolutionary inert, being neither conserved nor removed. Some pseudogenes, although not translated into protein, are at least transcribed into RNA [59-61]. In some cases these pseudogenes transcripts are capable for influencing the activity of other genes that code for proteins, therby altering expression and in turn affecting the phenotype of the organisms. Pseudogenes were first discovered in the 1970s

39

when acopy of 5sRNA gene was found in Xenopus laevis with homology to the active genes, but with a clear truncation that rendered it non functional [59]. Sciences sporadic discovery and characterizations of pseudogenes since from 20 years, which gave three classes of pseudogenes I) Unitary Pseudogenes, II) Duplicated Pseudogenes, III) Processed Pseudogenes (figure 5).

Figure 5. Types of Pseudogenes

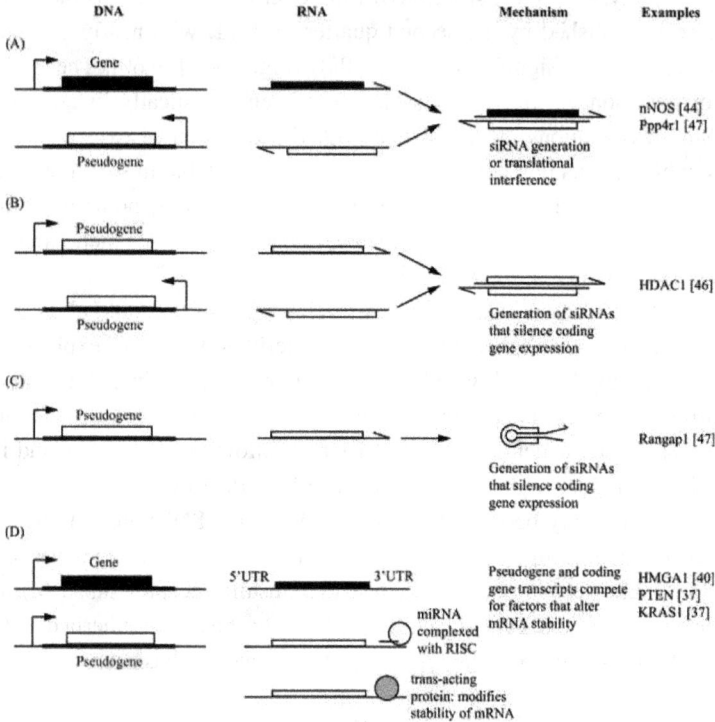

Unitary pseudogenes, they are formed when spontaneous mutation occur in a coding gene that abolish either transcription or translation, b) duplicated pseudogenes, it is formed when replication of the chromosome is performed incorrectly, c) processed pseudogene, it is formed when an mRNA molecule is reversed transcribed and integrated into a new location in the parental genome [59].

Recent technical advances in molecular biology have had a profound impact on biology and medicine. Various computer and information science methods are becoming more and more important in biomedical research. Variety of biological depositories with data of macromolecules like DNA (Deoxyribonucleic acid), RNA (Ribonucleic Acid) and Protein (amino acids) their sequences, structures, genes, their annotations and gene expression data are stored and available through WWW World Wide Web.

3D- Central Dogma

Introduction to molecular Biology:The Genome

Genome can be defined as genetic information of an organism; this information has been encoded of four letter A, G, T and C as a sequence. Structurally this information is stored in DNA (Deoxyribonucleic acid) molecules. This nucleotide comprises of 2-deoxyribose sugar, one or more phosphate groups and nitrogen containing base. Each strand, nucleotides are joined by a phosphodiester linkage between the 5' carbon of one deoxyribose group to the 3' carbon of the next. There are four types of bases used in DNA, adenine (A), guanine (G), cytosine (C), and Thymine (T). The genetic information is always read from the 5' end towards the 3' end of a DNA strand. The two strands are antiparallel in that the 5' end of one strand is connected with the 3' end of the other and vice versa.

The complementarity of the two strands lies in that an A in one strand will always be connected by two hydrogen bonds with a T in the opposite strand, and vice versa, and a C in one strand will always be connected by three hydrogen bonds with a G in the opposite strand, and vice versa.

The human genome contains approximately 3.1 billion base pairs packaged in chromosomes and located in the cell nucleus. There are 22 autosomes numbered 1-22 and two sex chromosomes X and Y. humans, as other higher organisms, are diploid meaning that (normally) all somatic cells, except red blood cells, which have no nucleus, have 23 pairs of chromosomes. Trisomies occur, but boost people have 22 pairs of autosomes (chromosomes 1-22). In addition, females have one pair of two X chromosomes, while males have one pair with one X chromosomes and one Y chromosome. Egg cells contain one copy of each of the 23 pairs of the female, while sperm cells contain one copy of each autosome and either one X chromosome or one Y chromosome.

Genes, RNA's and Proteins-

Genetic information is transferred from parent to offspring in unit of chromosomes, the basic unit of hereditary in the gene. Conceptually, genes are sequences of As, Cs, Gs and Ts containing the information required to synthesize specific proteins. "Proteins are the main catalysts, structural elements, signalling messengers and molecular machines of biological tissues" [62]. In other words protein are the molecules that effectuate most biological processes in the cells.

Protein molecules are linear polymers of amino acids connected by peptide bonds. There are 20 common amino acids with different chemical properties. In addition to the peptide bonds connecting each amino acid with the next, bonds may also be formed between amino acids on different parts of the polymer, giving rise to a three dimensional shape (conformation). The shape of protein is largely determined by the amino acid sequence, and in turns determines the chemical properties of the protein. Rather simplified, synthesis of biochemically active proteins consists of three steps: transcription, translation and protein folding. It should however be noted that some proteins are further modified, by, for instance, phosphorylation, glycosylation or bonding to other proteins or RNAs [63].

Protocol starts with when the DNA sequence of the gene is transcribed and an intermediate product called messenger ribonucleic acid (mRNA) molecule is synthesized by RNA polymerase enzymes. mRNA resemble single stranded DNA molecule but have the base uracil (U) in all positions where DNA would posses thymine (T). DNA transcription involves a complex machinery, but, roughly, starts when an RNA polymerase finds a start signal, proceeds in the 5' to 3' direction and ends at a stop signal. In this process one of the two DNA strands, the template strand, is copied into an RNA transcript that is equivalent (except for the U for T substitution) to the non- template strand. In humans and other higher eukaryotes, the raw RNAs are further processed by RNA- splicing producing mRNAs [64].

Second step of protein synthesis begins with when, mRNA are read linearly by ribosomes and transfer RNAs (tRNAs). A ribosome is a large complex of RNA and protein molecules that binds together mRNA with two tRNAs and catalyzes the formation of peptide bonds between neighbouring amino acids. The mRNA sequence is read in triplets called codons. With few exceptions, the 64 possible codons have a universal meaning across all species, each code for a unique amino acid or function as a stop signal (termination codon) for translation process. Those translated genetic code is carried out by tRNA molecules, which 'transport' the correct amino acid to the ribosome upon reading a given codon [65].

42

Last step before the protein reaches a functional form is folding from a linear polymer to a three dimensional structure. The structural shape or conformation of the protein determines its ability to react chemically and also helps to determine its function. Thus in order for all the cell to work correctly, it is necessary that the proteins fold correctly to the right conformation. unlike transcription and translation, protein folding does not follow a linear sequence of steps and the native structure of a protein is often but one of many physically possible conformations. However sometimes protein do not fold as they should, despite several corrections mechanisms. Misfolded proteins are normally digested before they can harm the cell.

Gene Expression and Function

Recent study says human genome contains somewhere between 30 to 40 thousands genes [64,65]. Far from all of these have been found, and still are under process for characterization. The genes range widely in length, from just a few hundred to several hundred thousands base pairs. Human genes comprises of both protein coding and non-coding regions called as exons and Introns. During splicing process, regions of the RNA transcript corresponding to introns are removed and exons corresponding regions are spliced to form mRNA. Many genes have alternate splice variants, implying that the same gene may give rise to more than one protein. Precise estimates of the number of distinct proteins in the human body are difficult to obtain, but recent results indicate that each gene, on average, has approximately three splice variants, implying that the there are over 90 thousand different proteins.

Gene Expression Diversity

Over 200 different cell types in the human body only three does not contain the same DNA. The vast majority of the cells contains the same set of genes but exhibit a highly diverse composition of proteins, accounting for the differences of function and structure between different cell types, and also between different states of the same cell. Thus, gene expression, or the rate at which the various proteins are produced, is the key to cell diversity. The number of active copies of a protein is regulated by several mechanisms: translational control, mRNA degradation control, Transcriptional Control, RNA processing control, and several modes of protein activity control [66]. The cell regulates the level of active copies of various proteins over time and in response to internal and external signals.

Gene and protein function

The most striking effects of gene function can be found in genes that are inherited in distinct variants, including non-functional, resulting in synthesis of different variants of the corresponding protein, or no protein to all. A number of genes are named and known by detrimental syndromes caused by their malfunctioning or other easily identified phenotypic traits linked to particular variants [64,65]. Many of these extreme cases in which the expression of the corresponding gene is not modulated by 'normal' mechanisms. In general, gene function, or more correctly, the biological effect of the corresponding product(s), is much more differentiated.

Protein functions and genes can be described along many dimensions [62,69,70]. Molecular biology says protein functions can be described in terms of structural class and which types of bond the molecule can form, also describes the interaction of protein with other protein and DNA i.e. Protein- Protein Interactions, and DNA-protein Interaction. Most proteins are involved in a limited number of cellular process.- for many protein only one and are thus spatially restructed to specific parts of the cell and temporally restricted to specific parts of the cell cycle. On another aspect protein can be classified according to what they 'do'. Whether they catalyze any chemical reactions, are part of any structural elements, is they bind to DNA or process any chemical signals, and so on. Finally proteins and genes may be classified according to their phenotypic effects [70].

The genes are themselves not biochemically active. Their biological importance and functions are effectuated by, and hence, derived from the function of their proteins. Indication of protein function can be found from protein structure and from the relative levels of protein species [70]. There are several limitations to protein based methods in the context of studying gene function on genome wide level [71]. For instance, current technologies to measure protein abundance are neither sufficiently high throughput no sufficiently accurate to obtain precise measurements for all protein present in complex biological samples, such as extracted from a cell. Since important parts of the control of gene expression is exerted on the mRNA level, valuable information about gene function can be obtained by measuring abundance of mRNA species. It should however, be kept in mind that many questions cannot be answered by studying gene expression alone-not even on the level of protein abundance.

To study co expression which is indicative of protein interaction but much more direct evidencecan be found from studies of protein structure and protein complexes.

Gene Database

Variety of Huge data, comprehensive collections of information about genes, proteins and their functionexists. Due to rapid progress in discovering and characterizing novel genes and proteins, the world wide web has become one of the primary source of up-to-date information. Listed there are few of the most central databases describes.

The Online Mendelian Inheritance in Man (OMIM) [72] database currently contains descriptions for 9,846 genes or phenotypic loci. This database, which "is a continuously updated catalog of human genes and genetic disorders", in only one of many databases containing descriptions of human genes andtheir biological roles.

The LocusLink [73] database is another comprehensive database with information about human genes, as well as other genetic loci in Homo sapiens and selected model organisms. Together with each locus, locus link provides, if known, information about the corresponding protein, function, phenotype links, etc. the database also provides meta-information pertaining to the status of its content as well as number of links to external data. In particular, each locus is linked to a number of sequence related resources, such as various chromosome maps and mRNA, protein and genomic sequence data.

The international nucleotide sequence database Collaboration comprising the three sister databases, Genbank [73-76], the EMBL nucleotide database, and DDBJ Japan organizes and avail DNAsequences publicly. Each sequence is stored in a separate record also containing annotations such as source, references, and biological features and qualifiers. The structural annotations follow a fixed format defined by the DDBJ/EMBL/Genbank Feature table.

Expressed sequence Tags (ESTs) are cDNA representations of fragments of expressed mRNA. Raw EST sequence data are collected in subdivisions of the nucleotide databases. Many ESTs can be linked to characterized genes are proteins, but a large number of ESTs cannot be identified forts [77-80] to provide order among the many ESTs that have been sequenced. The database contains 'clusters' of EST grouped by sequence similarity with each cluster putatively representing a unique gene.

Compared to the genomic sequence data, ESTs provide a much more direct link to proteins.When joined together into a full length mRNAs, ESTs can be used to predict novel proteins or mapped to characterized proteins. Various number of protein related (sequence and structure) databases are available. The PDB (protein databank) [81] maintained by the RCSB (Research Collaboratory for Structural Bioinformatics) is the primary source for protein structures. The SWISS PROT database [82] is a protein sequence database with an extensive level of annotation making it the de facto catalog of proteins for a number of organisms. The TrEMBL [83] supplement to SWISS-PROT contains a non redundant set of translations of all coding sequence in the EMBL nucleotide sequence database that do not correspond to existing SWISS-PROT entries.

Methods for mRNA detection

There are various method to detect mRNA levels. Some methods briefly described below, mRNA expression can be measured by for instance, Northern Blots, various methods based on the polymerase chain reaction (RT-PCR) [84-86], sequencing for cDNA-libraries [82,87], and serial analysis of gene expression (SAGE) [87-89]. Except for de novo cDNA sequencing, all methods used to measure mRNA require prior knowledge of the DNA sequence of the gens of interest. Thus, large-scale assays of gene expression are natural successors of comprehensive sequencing projects.

Most methods used to detect specific mRNA molecule rely on the fundamental principles of hybridization between complementary nucleic acids. This was discovered by first noting that duplex DNA will de- naturalize in aqueous solution when the temperature is raised to approximately 100 degrees celcius. The 'melting ' temperature depends on properties of both the sequence and solution. If the temperature is lowered, the single strands will re-naturalize (hybridize) to form stable duplexes again. Similar hybridization reactions can be obtained to form heteroduplexes with DNA and RNA, as well as to form homo-duplexes with two strands of RNA. The hybridization process will happen spontaneously if the single stranded nucleic acids are allowed to collide and stable and stable duplexes will be formed if there is sufficient base-pair complementarity, depending on the temperature. By adjusting the temperature (and other properties), it is possible to control the stringency and use hybridization to nucleic acids with known sequence (and identity) to interrogate very specifically biological samples with unknown composition of DNA or RNA.

Analysis of Gene Expression Data

Large scale screenings of gene expression levels have been applied in a number of biological settings [90]. These applications range in complexity from simple two –sample analyses in which the main question may be to identify differentially expressed genes to large clinically relevant screens of gene expression in upto hundred samples from patient derived tissues [91-94]. In the latter type of experiments, the goal is often to identify genes by whose expression levels it is possible to classify patients, or more generally samples, into relevant groups, for instance, to distinguish patients likely to survive or respond to a treatment from those who are not. Another type of experiment in which large- scale gene expression have been used in time course study. In this type of experiments the investigator aims to identify genes whose expression levels vary and co-vary across different time points after some reference state; the reference state could be the start of a cell cycle [95], some other point of time in the cell cycle in which cells are conveniently arrested, or immediately after a perturbation of the cell state, for instance, heat shock or drug treatment [96].

Cluster Methods

K- means

If there is reason to believe that the objects to be clustered belong to disjoint subclasses, hierarchical clustering methods may be less appropriate. The so called K-means and the more genereal K-mediad methods are clustering methods that naturally produce disjoint clusters. Briefly, the K-Means methodproceeds by the following steps:-

Decide upon a number K of clusters to find and initialize K clusters by defining K cluster Centers.Repeat until some pre-defined convergence criterion is reached:

For each data point (re-) assign it to the nearest cluster.

Update each cluster center as the centroid of all data points assigned to the corresponding cluster.

Other clustering Methods

Clustering is a fundamental way of data analysis. In addition to several variants and generalizations of the previously described methods, an interesting extension involves the simultaneous clustering along two dimensions, e.g., genes and samples. Relationships between subsets of genes and subset of samples can be found by clustering each dimension sequentially, but a combined simultaneous clustering along both axes may provide even more interesting relationships to be found. Recently at lest two strategies applied to gene expression data have been reported: coupled two way clustering [96,97] and biclustering [98].

Typical clustering methods can be described as global approaches, as they try to impose a structure on all observations in a dataset. Gene shaving is an iterative method that can be used to identifyinteresting subgroups without simultaneously clustering all objects [99]. One 'cluster' is singled out in each step and observations are allowed to belong to more than one cluster.

Supervised data analysis

Clustering and other unsupervised methods for data analysis can in one way be viewed merely as methods for data reduction or summarization- they can describe structure in the data but provide no explanation of the structure found. Incorporating prior knowledge into the analysis allows more directed studies to be conducted and stronger hypothesis may be tested.

In a simple two sample comparison, a natural first question is to identify genes whose expressiondiffers the most. As with other biological data, gene expressions are often converted to ratios in order to measure difference in terms of fold change. Often more than one sample is collected for each group, either by replication or by analysing material from several samples from each group. If such data are available, there are several statistical methods that could, and should, be used to identify those genes with the most interesting gene expression differences across the two groups. Essentially, the analysis proceeds by averaging the expression measurements within each group and comparing the averages. Rather than ranking the genes by differences according to significance. Several statistical tests are, available for these purposes [100,101].

In many studies there may be data from samples from more than two groups. If the experimentaldesign of the study is appropriate, an analysis of Variance (ANOVA) may be conducted.

In addition to assessing the levels of gene expression across groups of samples for the genes in a study, itis often of interest to assess whether such differences can be used to classify new samples. i.e., to use expression data in prediction. Some of the promises of such classification analyses lies in the possibility of using gene expression for classification of phenotypes, but it may also be possible to use gene expression to predict gene function of uncharacterized (functionally) transcripts. Already, there have been studies that have tried to classify genes according to level of expression in collecting of samples [102]. Several machine learning and statistical methods for predictive analyses are applicable to gene expression data given the existence of an a priori classification of the data.

Support Vector machines

The statistical learning theory formulated by Vapnik [103] introduces the support vector machine (SVM). The SVM method is conceptually simple approach for binary classification where the two classes are described by lying on either side of a hyper lane. Unlike Fisher's linear discriminate, the separating hyper lane is not calculated in the input space directly but in a higher dimensional space. SVMs have been used with good results on gene expression data [102].

Combined Approaches

Many interesting analyses of gene expression are studies combining unsupervised methodswith supervised methods, but, in particular and perhaps conceptually more interesting, studies combining analysis of gene expression data with external information, such as, for instance, sequence data, information from annotation databases, as well as, information extracted from the literature.

Based on the assumption that similarly expressed genes are regulated by the same, or similar, transcription factors, several studies have reported findings of plausible regulatory elements in groups of genes co clustered by gene expression data [104-106].

Text analysis for molecular biology

The amount of text data available in electronic form is rapidly growing. The transition from paper to digital media has revolutionized distribution and access to information –molecular biology and other biomedical sciences are no exceptions. Through the World Wide Web a growing number of scientific journals are publishing electronic versions online, sometimes even before the printed versions are available. However, timely and efficient access alone is not enough to use this information productively. Relevant information has to be correctly related to the problem at hand before it can be found and put to use. ***These issues have spurred a lot of research into retrieval and extraction of biomedical information, many motivated by challenges of interpreting expression measurements for thousands of genes***. Both information retrieval (IR) [107-108] and information extraction (IE) [109,110] rely on some form of special text analysis.

Briefly IR can be said to have the goal of returning a subset of relevant pieces of text from a larger set based on a user query, while IE can be said to have the goal of gathering occurrence of pre- specified pieces of information, such as descriptions of events or entities, from texts written in natural language.

Although important differences exist, the two fields are quite related, both with each other as well as with other research fields processing natural language.

Both IR and IE are commonly evaluated in terms of precision and recall. Precision is defined as the number of correct answers given by the system divided by the total numbers of answer given by the system. Recall is defined as the number of correct answers given by the system divided by the total number of correct answers. For IR, ans answer given by the system corresponds to a returned documents, and for IE, an answer corresponds to a detected occurrence. The correct answers correspond to relevant documents and actual occurrences for IR and IE, respectively. Other performance measures have also been used.

Various complex diseases like type 2 diabetes, obesity and cardiovascular diseases, multiple genetic and environmental factors as well as the interaction between these factors determine the phenotype. The contribution of genetic discoveries to the clinical management of diabetes and obesity remains limited to the small portion of cases with monogenic forms of disease [111]. The first is the modest effect size of the implicated variants. The common gene variants with the greatest effects on the risk of type 2 diabetes (TCF7L2 (transcription factor 7 like 2) in Europeans and KCNQ1 (Potassium Voltage Gated Channel Subfamily) in Asians) [111-113].

One of the obstacles to the translation of variants implicated in multifactorial form of Diabetes and obesity relates to the speed with which risk allele discovery has led to an improved understanding of the biological disease. Most alleles implicated in monogenic and syndromic forms of diabetes and obesity alter the coding sequence and therefore have dramatic and largely predictable effects on the function of the gene. The molecular diagnostics to derive clinically useful prognostic and therapeutic information relies on this relatively straightforward assignment of functional significance. However, most susceptibility genetic variants lie outside the coding regions of genes and are assumed to influence transcript regulation rather than gene function [112].

The worldwide rise in prevalence of type 2 diabetes and other cardio metabolic disorders has led to an intense search for genetic factors influencing the susceptibility for these common disorders. Although environmental influences, such as high-caloric fat- and carbohydrate-enriched diets and a sedentary lifestyle with markedly reduced physical activity, certainly accelerate disease development in those with genetic predisposition, it is nonetheless of great clinical importance, and indeed a formidable challenge, to elucidate the genetic variants that increase the risk of diseases like type 2 diabetes [114]. Even though much research has been conducted, the knowledge of the specific causes of common complex diseases at the genetic level is still somewhat at its infancy. More detailed insight into the genetic risk factors and the underlying molecular mechanisms involved in type 2 diabetes and related traits is expected to improve clinical investigations, advance the prevention of disease development, elucidate the diseases mechanisms and hopefully highlight new pathways relevant for therapeutic intervention.

3E-DIABETES MELLITUS and GENOMICS

Definition, description and classification of diabetes mellitus

Diabetes mellitus is a group of metabolic disorders of heterogeneous etiology characterized by persistent elevated blood glucose levels (hyperglycaemia) with disturbances of carbohydrate, fat and protein metabolism as a result of defects in insulin secretion, impaired effectiveness of insulin action, or both [115,116]. The increasing global prevalence of type 2 diabetes is tied to rising rate of obesity. The disease is classified as type 1 diabetes, type 2 diabetes, gestational diabetes and other types of diabetes, including monogenic diabetes [115]. Type 1 and type 2 diabetes are considered the two major types. Type 1 diabetes normally develops before adulthood and is typically caused by an auto-immune destruction of the insulin-producing ù-cells leading to an absolute insulin deficiency, whereas type 2 diabetes is normally associated with insulin resistance and relative insulin deficiency.

Diabetes is a major global health problem due to dramatically increasing prevalence in both the western world and in the developing countries. Rising health care costs are a serious problem, and a significant portion of health care spending is incurred by people with diabetes. The number of people with diabetes is increasing due to aging (increase in the proportion of people >65 years of age), general population growth, urbanization, and increasing prevalence of obesity and physical inactivity. The total number of people worldwide with diabetes is projected to rise from 285 million in 2010 to 439 million in 2030 corresponding to a predicted increase in prevalence from 6.4% in 2010 to 7.7% in 2030 [117]. Similar patterns are seen in Norway as well. Data from the

Nord - Trøndelag Health surveys (HUNT) indicate an increase in the prevalence of diabetes during the last two decades, with 3.8% of women and 4.9% of men being diagnosed with diabetes in 2006-08 [118]. The prevalence of diabetes is probably underestimated due to the rapid rise in the number of obese individuals. In Norway, studies have indicated that the total number of individuals with diabetes is twice of what has been diagnosed [119].

Diagnosing diabetes. The diagnostic criteria for diabetes and pre-diabetes (intermediate hyperglycaemia such as impaired fasting glucose (IFG) and impaired glucose tolerance (IGT)) have been debated for several years and modified numerous times. In 1997 the fasting glucose cut-off level was lowered from 7.8 to 7.0 mmol/l [116,120] and in 2003 the American Diabetes Association (ADA) changed the threshold for IFG from 6.1 to 5.6 mmol/l [121]. Moreover, since 2010, ADA included the use of glycated haemoglobin (HbA1c) to diagnose diabetes and to identify individuals at "increased risk for future diabetes" [115].

Table 1. Criteria for Diabetes Mellitus

	WHO 2006	ADA 2016
Diabetes Mellitus		
Fasting glucose	• 7.0 mmol/l	• 7.0 mmol/l
2-hour glucose	• 11.1 mmol/l	• 11.1 mmol/l
HbA1c	• 6.5 %	• 6.5 %
Non-diabetic hyperglycemia		
Fasting glucose	6.1 - 6.9 mmol/l	5.6 - 6.9 mmol/l
2-hour glucose	7.8 – 11.0 mmol/l	7.8 – 11.0 mmol/l
HbA1c	-	5.7 - 6.4 %

Present diagnostic criteria for diabetes, and non-diabetic hyperglycaemia (IFG and IGT) according to serum/plasma levels. Adapted from [115,122,123]. From a WHO consultation report from 2016 that was an addendum to the diagnostic criteria published in the 2006. Impaired fasting glucose. impaired glucose tolerance.

HbA1c levels are better predictors than fasting glucose of the development of long-term complications in type 1 and type 2 diabetes [124]. In addition, higher levels in the sub-diabetic range have been shown to predict type 2 diabetes risk and cardiovascular disease [125,126]. Thus, in a very recent report, the World Health Organization (WHO)

As well recommended the use of HbA1c in the diagnosis of diabetes [124]. The current diagnostic criteria for diabetes and intermediate hyperglycaemia according to WHO and ADA are shown in Table 1.

Type 2 diabetes is thought to be primarily heterogeneous and polygenic with low penetrance for the variants discovered, there exist monogenic types of non-autoimmune diabetes showing a Mendelian dominant pattern of inheritance, of which maturity-onset diabetes of the young (MODY) is the most common type [127]. Monogenic disorders of diabetes accounts for approximately 1-2% of all non-autoimmune diabetes and are largely affecting genes involved in ü-cell development and function [128]. The onset of disease usually occurs in childhood or young adulthood, generally before 25 years of age, although the hyperglycemia is mild in some cases and may be missed, as with type 2 diabetes. When hyperglycemia is detected in children, MODY may be misdiagnosed as type 1 diabetes. Genetic studies have defined a number of subtypes of MODY. Mutations in the genes encoding hepatic nuclear factor 4 (HNF4), glucokinase (GCK), hepatic nuclear factor 1 alpha and 1 beta (HNF1A and HNF1B), pancreatic and duodenal homeobox 1 (PDX1), transcription factor neurogenic differentiation 1 (NEUROD1), krüppel-like factor 11 (KLF11), transcription factor paired box 4 (PAX4), carboxyl ester lipase (CEL), insulin (INS) and B-lymphocyte specific tyrosine kinase (BLK) are the cause of the 11 known forms of MODY (MODY1-11) [129]. The most frequent forms of MODY results from mutations in the genes: HNF1A, GCK, HNF4A and HNF1B [130-132]. Other monogenic forms of diabetes include mitochondrial diabetes, neonatal diabetes, syndromes of severe insulin resistance and rare genetic syndromes. There are five genes currently known to be associated with non-syndromic permanent neonatal diabetes: potassium channel, inwardly rectifying, subfamily J, member 11 (KCNJ11), ATP- binding cassette, subfamily C, member 8 (ABCC8), INS, GCK, and pancreas/duodenum homeobox protein 1 (PDX1) [132-135]. Genetic testing and counseling is indicated and highly relevant when monogenic forms of diabetes are suspected, since patients with mutations in KCNJ11, ABCC8, HNF1A and HNF4A can be treated with oral antidiabetic agents (sulphonylureas) [136,137], in contrast to most of those who have mutations in the other genes. Prognosis, treatment and complications may also vary between the various forms of monogenic diabetes, depending on which gene that is affected. The predictive and clinical value of genetic testing is therefore substantial for monogenic forms of diabetes [127].

Type 2 Diabetes – Epidemiology, pathophysiology and long-term complications

An improved understanding of epidemiology, pathophysiology of type 2 diabetes can be achieved through genetic discovery provides new opportunities for treatment, diagnosis and monitoring (22,50), uptill now which is not fully understood, but presumably, type 2 diabetes develops when a diabetogenic lifestyle [138] (i.e. excessive caloric intake, inadequate caloric expenditure, obesity) acts in conjugation with a susceptible genotype. The majority of patients who develop type 2 diabetes are obese [139,140]. Energy-dense diet as a risk factor has, however, shown to be independent of baseline obesity for the development of type 2 diabetes [140]. Further, it has been suggested that type 2 diabetes in some cases are caused by environmental pollutants [142]. Even though there is some disparity regarding the reasons for the development of type 2 diabetes, most physicians and scientists agree that the major independent risk factors for developing type 2 diabetes are: obesity [143,144], family history of type 2 diabetes (first-degree relative) [145], ethnicity (some ethnic groups have higher prevalence of diabetes) [146,147], history of previous IGT or IFG [148], hypertension or dyslipidemia [149,150], physical inactivity [151], history of gestational diabetes [152], low birth weight as a result of an in utero environment [153], polycystic ovarian syndrome leading to insulin resistance [154], and finally, decline in insulin secretion due to advancing age [154,155]. Until recently, type 2 diabetes was considered to be a disease confined to adulthood, rarely observed in individuals under the age of 40, but clinically based reports and regional studies suggest that type 2 diabetes in children and adolescents is now more frequently being diagnosed [156,157]. This reflects the increasing number of children entering adulthood with unprecedented levels of obesity.

Type 2 diabetes is primarily caused by obesity, insulin resistance in liver, skeletal muscle and adipose tissue and a relative insulin secretion defect by the pancreatic ù-cell (116,117). Insulin is a hormone produced by the pancreatic ù-cells and is the key hormone for the regulation of blood glucose. The hormone stimulates uptake of glucose from the blood in the muscle and fat tissue, storage of glucose as glycogen in the liver and muscle cells, and uptake and esterification of fatty acids in adipocytes. In addition, insulin inhibits the breakdown of proteins, the hydrolysis of triglycerides and the production of glucose from amino acids, lactate and glycerol. Glucagon, which is also secreted by the endocrine pancreas, has the opposite effects to that of insulin. The hormone causes the liver to convert stored glycogen into glucose, thereby increasing blood glucose. Besides, glucagon stimulates insulin secretion, so that glucose can be used by insulin-dependent tissues. Hence, glucagon and insulin are part of a feedback system that keeps blood glucose at the right level.

Figure 6. Insulin production and action of diabetes mellitus.

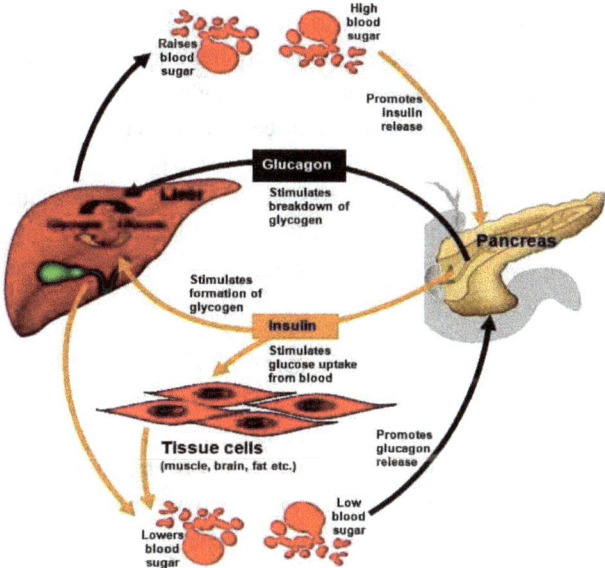

Insulin production and action. Diabetes results from an imbalance between the insulin-producing capacity of the pancreatic ü-cells and the requirement for insulin action in insulin target tissues such as liver, adipose tissue and skeletal muscle. Redrawn and modified after the IDF Diabetes Atlas [155].

For type 2 diabetes to occur the balanced relationship between insulin action and release have tobe disrupted. In other words, type 2 diabetes develops mainly in those who cannot increase insulin secretion sufficiently to compensate for their insulin resistance. Whereas insulin resistance is an early phenomenon partly related to obesity, pancreas ü-cell function declines gradually over time already before the onset of clinical hyperglycemia. Several mechanisms have been proposed for these two defects. Insulin resistance have been ascribed to elevated levels of free fatty acids [158], inflammatory cytokines [159], adipokines [160] and mitochondrial dysfunction [161], while glucose toxicity [162], lipotoxicity [163], and amyloid formation [164] have been proposed as central aspects for ü-cell dysfunction [165).

The medical and socioeconomic burden of type 2 diabetes is generally caused by the associated complications of the disease. The severe complications accompanying type 2 diabetes are mostly microvascular (e.g. retinopathy, neuropathy and nephropathy) and macrovascular diseases, leading to reduced quality of life and increased morbidity and mortality from end-stage renal failure and cardiovascular disease (CVD). Hyperglycemia plays a central role in the development and progression of the vascular complications, which often persist and progress despite improved glucose control,possibly as a result of prior occurrences of hyperglycemia. Increased cardiovascular risk, however, appears to begin before the development of frank hyperglycemia, presumably because of the effects of insulin resistance. This phenomenon has been described as the "ticking clock" hypothesis of complications [166,167], where the clock starts ticking for microvascular risk at the onset of hyperglycemia, and for macrovascular risk at some antecedent point, i.e. with the onset of insulin resistance.

It is generally accepted that the long-term complications of diabetes mellitus are far less common and less severe in people who have well-controlled blood sugar levels [168,169]. However, some recent trails that had great success in lowering blood sugar in type 2 diabetes patients, but no success in reducing deaths from cardiovascular disease, challenges the theory of hyperglycemia as the major cause of diabetic complications [170]. The familial clustering of the degree and type of diabetic complications indicates that genetics may also play a role in causing diabetic complications [171,172]. Although not fully understood, the complex mechanisms by which diabetes leaDiabetic to these complications involves hyperglycemia and both functional and structural abnormalities of small blood vessels along with accelerating factors such as smoking, elevated.

GENETIC PREDISPOSITION AND SUSCEPTIBILITY GENES FOR TYPE 2 DIABETES AND DIABETES RELATED TRAITS

Heritability of type 2 diabetes

Type 2 Diabetes (T2D) is a complex disease that is caused by a complex interplay between genetic, epigenetic and environmental factors. While the major environmental factors, diet and activity level, are well known, identification of those genetic factors has been a challenge. (173).

Phenotypic variation among individuals may be attributable to genetics, environmental challenge and/or random events. Heritability is the proportion of phenotypic variation in a population that is due to genetic variation between individuals. Heritability of a trait or condition is often estimated on the basis of parent-offspring correlations for continuous traits or the ratio of the incidence in first-degree relatives of affected persons to the incidence in first-degree relatives of unaffected persons. Heritability is also frequently estimated by comparing resemblances between twins.

The clinical assessment of type 2 diabetes has often incorporated genetic information in the form of family history. Although very simple, family information has helped to raise clinical awareness for an individual patient's risk of type 2 diabetes due to the strong heritability of this disease. In contrast to a population risk of ~7%, family studies have estimated that the risk for type 2 diabetes among offspring is, respectively, 3.5-fold and 6-fold higher for those with a single diabetic parent and two diabetic parents compared with offspring without parental diabetes [174]. Furthermore, the higher concordance rate of type 2 diabetes in monozygotic versus dizygotic twins and the high prevalence of type 2 diabetes in specific ethnic groups such as Pima Indians and Mexican Americans, all lend support to the existence of genetic determinants for type 2 diabetes [175]. Overall, estimates have shown that 30%–70% of type 2 diabetes risk can be ascribed to genetics [176]. It is also evident, for example from a recent study in Finnish families, that type 2 diabetes-related intermediate and quantitative traits show substantial heritability [177,178]. The patterns of inheritance therefore suggest that type 2 diabetes and its related traits are both polygenic and heterogeneous; hence multiple genes are involved and different combinations of genes play a role in different subsets of individuals. How many risk genes that exist and what their relative contributions are, remains somewhat uncertain. However, recent advances in genetic mapping of complex diseases have provided some information or at least great optimism in the dissection of the complex architecture of polygenic diseases such as type 2 diabetes.

Genetics of type 2 diabetes and intermediary phenotypes

Type 2 diabetes (T2D) is a complex disease that is caused by a complex interplay between genetic, epigenetic and environmental factors. (173). In the past 10-15 years, huge resources have been devoted to finding type 2 diabetes genes. These efforts have included many candidate-gene studies and extensive efforts to fine-map linkage signals. Linkage analysis and subsequent positional fine-mapping of candidates have been mostly inconclusive, despite the detection of multiple genomic regions putatively linked to diabetes [178]. There is one notable exception, namely transcription factor 7-like 2 genes (TCF7L2). In 2006, the Icelandic company decode Genetics identified a common type 2 diabetessusceptibility variant in the TCF7L2 gene region [179]. This result was interesting for two reasons. First,the variants that were found to alter risk did not explain the linkage signal, even though the investigators analyzed more than 200 markers across the region. This suggested that a non-candidate-gene or region- based association approaches, such as a GWAS, could have a great potential. Second, TCF7L2 was a completely unexpected gene, thus demonstrating that a genome-wide approach could uncover previously unknown disease pathways [180].

Variants in many candidate genes were extensively studied by association studies in the pre- GWA era. In most instances, however, the initial association was not replicated in subsequent analyses. The candidate gene studies produced more unequivocal evidence for common variants involved in type2 diabetes than did the linkage approach. The most robust candidate variants were the E23K variant in the KCNJ11 gene [181-183], the P12A variant in the peroxisome proliferator-activated receptor-Û(PPARG) gene [184], and common variation in the HNF1B and the Wolfram syndrome 1 (WFS1) genes [185,186]. Rare mutations in all of these four genes are causing monogenic forms of diabetes [187-190], and two are targets of anti- diabetic therapies. KCNJ11 encodes a component of a potassium channelwith a key role in û-cell physiology that is a target for the sulphonylurea class of drugs, and PPARG encodes a transcription factor involved in adipocyte differentiation that is a target for thethiazolodinedione class of drugs [175,178].

In the spring of 2007, the results from the first wave of GWA studies investigating type 2 diabetes genes were published, namely the French, decode, DGI, WTCCC and FUSION studies [191- 195]. These five independent GWA studies were all conducted using a two-stage strategy consisting of aGWA screen in an initial cohort of unrelated cases and controls followed by replication of the most significant findings in additional patients series. The initial GWAS were subsequently followed by five smaller GWA studies [196-201]. The screening and replication sets consisted primarily of European Whites, with the exception of the decode study which contained groups of Chinese and West Africans. Each of these early GWA studies of type 2 diabetes identified numerous potential susceptibility variants,but no less than nine loci emerged as being consistently associated with risk of type 2 diabetes across multiple studies. The nine loci were TCF7L2, solute carrier family 30, member 8 (SLC30A8), hematopoietically expressed homoeobox (HHEX), CDK5 regulatory subunit-associated protein 1-like 1 (CDKAL1), cyclin-dependent kinase inhibitor 2A/2B (CDKN2A/B), insulin-like growth factor 2 mRNA-binding protein 2 (IGF2BP2), fat mass- and obesity-associated gene (FTO), KCNJ11 and PPARG, among which three (TCF7L2, KCNJ11 and PPARG) had previously been implicated in type 2 diabetes.

The TCF7L2 gene is the most important type 2 diabetes susceptibility gene found to date [174]. Since its discovery, the association has been replicated in a variety of studies in subjects of different ethnicities [202-207]. In the U.K. population, the allelic odds ratio (OR) for the lead SNP (rs7903146, risk-allele frequency = 30%) is 1.36 and individuals carrying two risk (T) alleles are at nearly twice the risk of type 2 diabetes as are those with none [208]. The population attributable risk (PAR) is on theother hand somewhat lower, and varies with the variants' frequency in the population. TCF7L2 encodesa transcription factor in the Wnt-signaling pathway, which induces transcription of a number of genes, including pro glucagon, in the intestine. Recent studies have shown that there is an increased expression of TCF7L2 in the islets of pancreas in type 2 diabetes, which in turn results in impaired glucose- stimulated insulin secretion.

One of the most interesting regions to emerge from the first wave of GWAS for type 2 diabetes and CVD lies in a gene desert ~130 kb upstream of the CDKN2B gene on chromosome 9p21. Several SNPs in the 9p21 interval have demonstrated strong associations with coronary artery disease/myocardial infarction (MI) [209-212] and other vascular diseases such as stroke and intracranial and abdominal aneurisms [210-213]. All these SNPs are highly correlated (r2 >0.8) and found in a ~60 kb LD-block. The 9p21 region also contains two adjacent, but distinct type 2 diabetes signals separated by a recombination hotspot; a strong signal mapped to an 11 kb LD-block (represented by rs10811661) and a second signal (rs564398) located ~100 kb in a telomeric direction from the type 2 diabetes- associated interval [214-216]. After the initial GWASs, several studies have confirmed the association with the implicated candidate SNPs in type 2 diabetes [217-220] and CVD [221-225] and extended the number of CVD phenotypes associated with the region [226-230]. This raised the possibility of a shared genetic or mechanistic link causing both CVD and diabetes within this region. In support, a significant interaction was found between poor glycemic control and a variant within the 9p21 region on the risk of coronary heart disease in patients with type 2 diabetes [232]. However, the effects of the disease susceptibility variants for the two major disease loci have shown to be independent, since type 2 diabetesrisk variants do not seem to confer increased risk of cardiovascular disease or the other way around [233,234].

The risk variants identified in the 9p21 interval by GWAS are in general located in non-coding regions, since most reported risk variants do not appear in mature transcripts, and there are no known micro-RNAs mapping to this region [235]. This suggests that their effects probably are mediated by influences on gene expression of nearby genes in cis. Besides the coding sequences for the two cyclin- dependent kinase inhibitors, CDKN2A (p16INK4a) including its alternative reading frame (ARF) transcript variant (p14ARF), and CDKN2B (p15INK4b), the region contains a large anti-sense non- coding RNA gene, designated CDKN2BAS (formerly termed ANRIL). Recent studies have shown that expression of these genes is co-regulated and that most of the confirmed risk variants are all correlated with CDKN2BAS expression, indicating that CDKN2BAS could play a role in CDKN2B regulation [236]. Hence, modulation of CDKN2BAS expression may mediate susceptibility to several important diseases.

The individual SNP rs10757278 has been highlighted as a potential causal variant for the association with coronary artery disease based on effects on expression of the INK4/ARF locus (p15INK4b, p16INK4a, ARF and CDKN2BAS) [237]. Moreover, the rs10757278 SNP have also been mapped to one of 33 newly identified enhancers in the 9p21 interval, in which the risk variant disrupts atranscription factor binding site, thus having functional relevance for an atherosclerosis-associated pathway in human endothelial cells [238].

The French GWA study, one of the first five GWA studies investigating type 2 diabetes genes, involved non-obese diabetics and revealed that a version of a gene encoding a protein that transportszinc in the pancreas, SLC30A8, increased the risk of type 2 diabetes [208]. Of all the new type 2 diabetes genes discovered by the GWA approach, SLC30A8 are one of the few involving a non- synonymous polymorphism – an arginine to tryptophan substitution at amino acid 325. SLC30A8 has also recently been identified as an auto-antigen in human type 1 diabetes [239]. In contrast to SLC30A8, most of the genes identified in the GWA screens would not be considered typical candidate genes for type 2 diabetes and in most cases the variants are located in non-coding regions in or near the gene.

In the first wave of GWAS, all studies had relatively small sample sizes and were therefore to some extent statistically underpowered to detect variants with modest effect sizes. In recognition of this, data from three GWA studies were combined by the DIAGRAM consortium. Through meta-analysis comprising 10,128 individuals of European descent and ~2 million SNPs directly genotyped or imputed, followed by large-scale replication in up to 53,975 individuals, six additional type 2 diabetes susceptibility genes (JAZF1, CDC123, TSPAN8, THADA, ADAMTS9, and NOTCH2) were detected [240]. The initial GWA scans were mainly performed in cases and controls from European populations. For this reason GWA scans in other populations were warranted. The first GWA studies performed in Asian subjects with type 2 diabetes discovered a new gene, KCNQ1, which has later also been confirmed in European subjects [241,242]. Furthermore, a single GWA study in Taiwanese demonstrated genome-wide associations with type 2 diabetes for two other loci, SRR and PTPRD [243]. Notably, most type 2 diabetes variants have been shown to have an impact on pancreatic ü-cell function with a primary effect on insulin secretion rather than on insulin action [244]. A GWA study performed in French and Danish subjects revealed, however, a variant in the IRS1 gene, which together with PPARG being one of a limited number of type 2 diabetes loci so far displaying a diabetogenic potential through affecting peripheral insulin sensitivity [245].

The GWA approach has further demonstrated that genetic studies of glycemic traits can identify type 2 diabetes risk loci. Follow-up signals for type diabetes from GWA scans for fasting glucose or insulin secretion revealed from 2008 to 2010 a whole new set of type 2 diabetes susceptibility loci. The melatonin-receptor gene (MTNR1B), which highlights the link between circadian and metabolic regulation [172], was found to be associated with levels of fasting glucose and risk of type 2 diabetes [246-249]. Follow-up signals of a fourth GWA scan for fasting glucose identified, in addition to MTNR1B, five other loci (ADCY5, PROX1, GCK, GCKR and DGKB) associated with type 2 diabetes [176]. Very recently, several studies have reported even larger meta-analyses of GWA data from both European and Asian ethnic groups, leading to the identification of several new loci for type 2 diabetes, including RBMS1, DUSP9, KLF14, ARAP1, HMGA2, HNF1A, GRB14, ST6GAL1, VPS26A, HMG20A, AP3S2 and HNF4A [250-253]. Of these new loci, genetic and gene expression studies had previously suggested an important role for KLF14 in metabolic disease. A recent study demonstrated a network of genes whose expression was associated with KLF14 variation in trans, providing a framework for understanding how KLF14 influences disease risk [254]. Moreover, confirmation of a common variant associations at HNF1A and HNF4A [255,256] added new loci to those known to harbor both rare mutations causing monogenic forms of diabetes and common variants predisposing to multifactorial diabetes. The number is now 7, the others being PPARG, KCNJ11, WFS1, HNF1B and GCK.

Advances in genomic technology have initiated a myriad of novel genetic discoveries including more tan 2,000 common variants contributing to risk of complex disease. Overall, the power of genome- wide association studies, in combination with larger data sets, meta-analyses of the initial GWA studies, establishments of larger consortia (e.g. DIAGRAM, GIANT, MAGIC), GWA scans conducted on intermediary diabetes phenotypes (e.g. fasting glucose) and the use of study samples of different ethnicities, have delivered a whole set of new susceptibility loci for type 2 diabetes over the last five years, now counting around 50 loci [126,257]. The validated susceptibility loci along with their discovery method, cellular function and putative intermediary mechanism in diabetes are summarized in Table 2. The last reported type 2 diabetes susceptibility regions are individually only associated with a marginally increased risk for diabetes (OR<1.1), and can together explain only ~10% of the heritability seen for type 2 diabetes [258]. Clinical factors seem to predict the risk of diabetes development better than a sample of 16 genotyped type 2 diabetes associated SNPs, either alone or in combination [259].The clinical utility of the genome wide association studies is therefore controversial and have beenhighly debated [260-262].

Table 2. Showing the list of common SNPs (Single nucleotide Polymorphism) studied in Type IIDiabetes Mellitus

Sr.No	T2D RiskSNP	Gene/Nearest Gene	Gene Location	Chr	RA	OA	OR	TRAIT	Refs.
1	rs17106184	FAF1	intron	1	G	A	1.1	T2D	[70]
2	rs2296172	MACF1	coding -missense	1	G	A	1.1	2D	[79]
3	rs10923931	NOTCH2	intron	1	T	G	1.13	T2D	[4,80]
4	rs340874	PROX1	intergenic	1	C	T	1.07	Fasting glucose/HOMA B/T2D	[81]
5	rs243021	BCL11A	intergenic	2	A	G	1.08	T2D	[25]
6	rs243088	BCL11A	intergenic	2	T	A	1.07	T2D	[62]
7	rs2975760	CAPN10	intron	2	C	T	1.17	T2D	[48,82]
8	rs3792267	CAPN10	intron	2	G	A	1.17	T2D	[48,82]
9	rs7607980	COBLL1	coding-missense	2	T	C	1.14	T2D	[79]
10	rs560887	G6PC2/ABCB11	intron	2	T	C	1.03	Fasting glucose/T2D/HOMA B	[81]
11	rs780094	GCKR	intron	2	C	T	1.06	T2D/Fasting glucose/beta- cell function/triglycerides/fasting insulin	[81]
12	rs3923113	GRB14	intergenic	2	A	C	1.07	T2D	[62,65]
13	rs13389219	GRB14	intergenic	2	C	T	1.07	T2D	[62]

#	SNP	Gene	Location	Chr	Allele	Allele	OR	Phenotype	Ref
14	rs2943641	IRS1	intergenic	2	C	T	1.19	Fasting glucose/T2D/HOMAB, HOMA IR/AUC ins/AUC ratio/ISI	[83]
15	rs7578326	KIAA1486/IRS1	intron of uncharacterized LOC646736	2	A	G	1.11	T2D	[25]
16	rs7593730	RBMS1/ITGB6	intronic	2	C	T	1.11	T2D	[84]
17	rs7560163	RND3	intergenic	2	G	C	1.33	T2D	[67]
18	rs7578597	THADA	coding-missense	2	T	C	1.15	T2D	[4,80]
19	rs10200833	THADA	intron	2	G	C	1.06	T2D	[80,85]
20	rs6723108	TMEM163	intergenic	2	T	G	1.31	Decreased fasting plasma insulin/HOMA-IR/T2D	[74]
21	rs998451	TMEM163	intron	2	G	A	1.56	Decreased fasting plasma insulin/HOMA-IR/T2D	[74]
22	rs4607103	ADAMTS9-AS2	intron	3	C	T	1.09	T2D	[4,80]
23	rs6795735	ADAMTS9-AS2	intron	3	C	T	1.09	T2D	[4,80]

	rs ID	Gene	Location	Chr	Allele	Allele	OR	Phenotype	Ref
24	rs11708067	ADCY5	intron	3	A	G	1.12	T2D/2hr glucose/HOMAB	[81,86]
25	rs2877716	ADCY5	intron	3	C	T	1.12	2 h insulin adjusted for 2 h glucose/2 h glucose/T2D	[81,86]
26	rs11071657	FAM148B	intergenic	3	A	G	1.03	Fasting glucose/T2D/HOMA B	[81]
27	rs4402960	IGF2BP2	intron	3	T	G	1.11	T2D	[59]
28	rs1470579	IGF2BP2	intron	3	C	A	1.15	T2D	[26,59,72,87]
29	rs6808574	LPP	intergenic	3	C	T	1.07	T2D	[70]
30	rs1801282	PPARG	coding-missense	3	C	G	1.09	T2D	[59]
31	rs13081389	PPARG	intergenic	3	A	G	1.24	T2D	[25,53,59,87]
32	rs17036160	PPARG	intron	3	C	T	1.11	T2D	[85]
33	rs1797912	PPARG	intron	3	A	C	1.06	T2D	[85]
34	rs831571	PSMD6	intergenic	3	C	T	1.09	T2D	[63]
35	rs7647305	SFRS10	intergenic	3	C	T	1.08	BMI/obesityT2D	[88]
36	rs16861329	ST6GAL1	intron	3	G	A	1.09	T2D	[65]
37	rs6780569	UBE2E2	intergenic	3	G	A	1.21	T2D	[73]
38	rs6815464	MAEA	intron	4	C	G	1.13	T2D	[63]
39	rs7656416	MAEA	intron	4	C	T	1.15	T2D	[63,64]
40	rs6813195	TMEM154	intergenic	4	C	T	1.08	T2D	[70]
41	rs10010131	WFS1	intron	4	G	A	1.14	T2D	[4,89]
42	rs4689388	WFS1	nearGene-5	4	T	C	1.16	T2D	[83]
43	rs6446482	WFS1	intron	4	G	C	1.11	T2D	[25,89,90]

#	SNP	Gene	Function		Allele 1	Allele 2	OR	Trait	References
44	rs1801214	WFS1	coding-missense	4	T	C	1.13	T2D	[25,89,90]
45	rs459193	ANKRD55	intergenic	5	G	A	1.08	T2D	[62]
46	rs702634	ARL15	intron	5	A	G	1.06	T2D	[70]
47	rs4457053	ZBED3	intron of ZBED3-AS1	5	G	A	1.08	T2D	[25]
48	rs1048886	C6orf57	coding-missense	6	G	A	1.54	T2D	[91]
49	rs7754840	CDKAL1	intron	6	C	G	1.17	T2D	[25,27,59,60,66,73,92,93]
50	rs7756992	CDKAL1	intron	6	G	A	1.2	T2D	[27]
51	rs2206734	CDKAL1	intron	6	T	C	1.2	T2D	[25,27,59,60,66,73,92,93]
52	rs4712523	CDKAL1	intron	6	G	A	1.27	T2D	[25,27,59,60,66,73,83,92,93]
53	rs10946398	CDKAL1	intron	6	C	A	1.12	T2D	[25,27,59,60,66,73,92,93]
54	rs7766070	CDKAL1	intron	6	A	C	1.23	T2D	[25,27,59,60,66,73,92,93]
56	rs1535500	KCNK16	coding-missense	6	T	G	1.08	T2D	[63]
57	rs3130501	POU5F1-TCF19	nearGene-5	6	G	A	1.07	T2D	[70]
58	rs9505118	SSR1-RREB1	intron	6	A	G	1.06	T2D	[70]
59	rs9470794	ZFAND3	intron	6	C	T	1.12	T2D	[63]
60	rs17168486	DGKB	intergenic	7	T	C	1.15	T2D	[62]
61	rs2191349	DGKB/TMEM195	intergenic	7	T	G	1.06	Fasting glucose, Homa B/T2D	[81]

#	SNP	Gene	Region	Chr	Allele	Allele	OR	Trait	Reference
62	rs6467136	GCC1-PAX4	intergenic	7	G	A	1.11	T2D	[63]
63	rs4607517	GCK	intergenic	7	A	G	1.07	Fasting glucose/T2D/HOMA B	[81]
64	rs864745	JAZF1	intron	7	T	C	1.1	T2D	[4,80]
65	rs849134	JAZF1	intron	7	A	G	1.13	T2D	[25,80]
66	rs12113122	JAZF1	intron	7	G	C	1.55	T2D	[85]
67	rs972283	KLF14	intergenic	7	G	A	1.07	Reduced insulin sensitivity T2D	[25]
68	rs516946	ANK1	intron	8	C	T	1.09	T2D	[62]
69	rs515071	ANK1	intron	8	G	A	1.18	T2D Reduced beta-cell function	[62,64]
70	rs13266634	SLC30A8	coding-missense	8	C	T	1.19	T2D	[58]
71	rs11558471	SLC30A8	UTR-3	8	A	G	1.15	Fasting glucose, HOMA B T2D	[25,58,59,81,87,92,93]
72	rs3802177	SLC30A8	UTR-3	8	G	A	1.26	T2D	[25,58,59,81,87,92,93]
73	rs896854	TP53INP1	intron	8	T	C	1.06	T2D	[25]
74	rs10965250	CDKN2A/2B	intergenic	9	G	A	1.2	T2D	[25,27,59,60,66,73,92,93]
75	rs2383208	CDKN2A/2B	intergenic	9	A	G	1.19	T2D	[25,27,59,60,66,73,92,93]
76	rs7018475	CDKN2A/2B	intergenic	9	G	T	1.35	T2D	[25,27,59,6066,73,92,93]
77	rs564398	CDKN2A/2B	intergenic	9	T	C	1.12	T2D	[25,27,59,60,66,73,92,93]

#	rs ID	Gene	Location	Chr			OR	Trait	Ref
78	rs10757282	CDKN2A/2B	intergenic	9	C	T	1.14	T2D	[25,27,59,60,66,73,92,93]
79	rs10811661	CDKN2B	intergenic	9	T	C	1.2	T2D	[25,59,60,66,68,80,87,92]
80	rs7034200	GLIS3	intron	9	A	C	1.03	Fasting glucose/T2D/HOMA B	[81]
81	rs7041847	GLIS3	intron	9	A	G	1.1	T2D	[63,66]
82	rs10814916	GLIS3	intron	9	C	A	1.11	T2D	[63,66,81]
83	rs17584499	PTPRD	intron	9	T	C	1.57	T2D	[95]
84	rs2796441	TLE1	intergenic	9	G	A	1.07	T2D	[62]
85	rs13292136	TLE4 (CHCHD9)	intergenic	9	C	T	1.11	T2D	[25]
86	rs553668	ADRA2A	UTR-3	10	A	G	1.42	T2D	[96]
87	rs10885122	ADRA2A	intergenic	10	G	T	1.04	Fasting glucose/HOMA B/T2D	[81]
88	rs12779790	CDC123, CAMK1D	intergenic	10	G	A	1.11	T2D	[4,80]
89	rs11257655	CDC123/CAMK1D	intergenic	10	C	T	1.15	T2D	[66,69,80]
90	rs10906115	CDC123/CAMK1D	intergenic	10	A	G	1.13	T2D	[66,69,80]
91	rs10886471	GRK5	intron	10	C	T	1.12	T2D	[66]
92	rs5015480	HHEX	intergenic	10	C	T	1.13	T2D	[25,58,59,92,93]
93	rs1111875	HHEX/IDE	intergenic	10	C	T	1.13	T2D	[59]
94	rs7903146	TCF7L2	intronic/promoter	10	T	C	1.35	T2D, fasting glucose,,2 h glucose	[51]

#	rs	Gene	Location	Chr			OR	Trait	Ref
95	rs4506565	TCF7L2	intron	10	T	A	1.34	Fasting glucose, HOMA B T2D	[25,27,51,58–61,80,87,92,93,97–99]
96	rs7901695	TCF7L2	intron	10	C	T	1.37	T2D	[25,27,51,58–61,80,87,92,93,97–99]
97	rs1802295	VPS26A	UTR-3	10	A	G	1.08	T2D	[65]
98	rs12571751	ZMIZ1	intron	10	A	G	1.08	T2D	[62]
99	rs11603334	ARAP1	UTR-5	11	G	A	1.13	T2D fasting proinsulin levels/fasting glucose/	[100]
100	rs1552224	CENTD2	intergenic	11	A	C	1.14	T2D	[25]
101	rs11605924	CRY2	intron	11	A	C	1.04	Fasting glucose/HOMA B/T2D	[81]
102	rs174550	FADIABETIC1	intron	11	T	C	1.04	Fasting glucose/T2D/HOMA B	[81]
103	rs2334499	HCCA2	intergenic	11	T	C	1.35	T2D	[101]
104	rs3842770	INS-IGF2	intron	11	A	G	1.18	T2D - African American	[94]
105	rs5219	KCNJ11	coding-missense	11	T	C	1.14	T2D	[54,59,60,87,99]
106	rs5215	KCNJ11	coding-missense	11	C	T	1.14	T2D	[54,59,60,87,99]
107	rs2237895	KCNQ1	intron	11	C	T	1.45	T2D	[71]
108	rs231362	KCNQ1	intron	11	G	A	1.08	T2D	[25]
109	rs163184	KCNQ1	intron	11	G	T	1.22	T2D	[62,71]

#	SNP	Gene	Location	Chr			OR	Phenotype	Reference
110	rs2237892	KCNQ1	intron	11	C	T	1.25	Reduced beta-cell function T2D	[25,71,72,92,95]
111	rs105501320	MADD	intron	11	G	C	1.01	T2D fasting proinsulin levels/fasting glucose	[100]
112	rs10830963	MTNR1B	intron	11	G	C	1.09	T2D	[102]
113	rs1387153	MTNR1B	intergenic	11	T	C	1.09	Reduced beta-cell function T2D	[25,95,102]
114	rs7138803	BCDIN3D/FAIM2	intergenic	12	A	G	1.11	BMI/obesity T2D	[88,103]
115	rs11063069	CCND2	intergenic	12	G	A	1.12	T2D	[62]
116	rs1153188	DCD	intergenic	12	A	T	1.08	T2D	[80]
117	rs1531343	HMGA2	intron of pseudogene	12	C	G	1.1	T2D	[25]
118	rs9668162	HMGA2	intron	12	G	C	1.26	T2D	[85]
119	rs7305618	HNF1A	intergenic	12	C	T	1.14	T2D	[25,68]
120	rs35767	IGF1	nearGene-5	12	G	A	1.04	Fasting insulin/T2D/HOMA IR	[81]
121	rs10842994	KLHDC5	intergenic	12	C	T	1.1	T2D	[62]
122	rs4275659	MPHOSPH9	intron	12	C	T	1.06	T2D	[70]
123	rs7957197	OASL/TCF1/HNF1A	intron of OASL	12	T	A	1.07	T2D	[25]
124	rs7961581	TSPAN8, LGR5	intergenic	12	C	T	1.09	T2D	[4,80]
125	rs9552911	SGCG	intron	13	G	A	1.63	T2D	[104]

#	rs ID	Gene	Region	Chr	Allele 1	Allele 2	OR	Phenotype	Ref
126	rs1359790	SPRY2	intergenic	13	G	A	1.15	T2D	[69]
127	rs2028299	AP3S2	UTR-3	15	C	A	1.1	T2D	[65]
128	rs7172432	C2CD4A/B	intergenic	15	A	G	1.14	Reduced beta-cell function, T2D	[73]
129	rs7178572	HMG20A	intergenic	15	A	G	1.09	lean T2D	[65,93]
130	rs7177055	HMG20A	intergenic	15	A	G	1.08	T2D	[62]
131	rs8042680	PRC1	intron	15	A	C	1.07	T2D	[25]
132	rs7403531	RASGRP1	intron	15	T	C	1.1	T2D	[66]
133	rs4502156	VPS13C/C2CD4A/B	intergenic	15	T	C	1.07	fasting proinsulin levels T2D	[100]
134	rs11634397	ZFAND6	intergenic	15	G	A	1.06	T2D	[25]
135	rs7202877	BCAR1	intergenic	16	T	G	1.12	T2D	[62]
136	rs8050136	FTO	intron	16	A	C	1.17	Increased BMI, reduced insulin sensitivity, T2D	[25,60,61,80,87,93,99,105]
137	rs9939609	FTO	intron	16	A	T	1.25	T2D (obese)	[25,60,61,80,87,93,99,105]
138	rs11642841	FTO	intron	16	A	C	1.13	T2D	[25,60,61,80,87,93,99,105]
139	rs4430796	HNF1B	intron	17	G	A	1.19	Reduced beta-cell function T2D	[66,106-108]
140	rs7501939	HNF1B	intron	17	T	C	1.09	T2D	[106]
141	rs391300	SRR	intron	17	G	A	1.28	T2D	[95]
142	rs4523957	SRR	nearGene-5	17	T		1.27	T2D	[95]
143	rs8090011	LAMA1	intron	18	G	C	1.13	lean T2D	[93]
144	rs17782313	MC4R	intergenic	18	C	T	1.06	BMI/T2D	[88,103]

145	rs12970134	MC4R	intergenic	18	A	G	1.08	T2D/BMI/waist circumference/insulin resistance	[62,109]
146	rs3794991	GATAD2A/CILP2	intron, intergenic	19	T	C	1.12	T2D	[62,85]
147	rs8108269	GIPR	intergenic	19	G	T	1.05	T2D	[62]
148	rs3786897	PEPD	intron	19	A	G	1.1	T2D	[63]
149	rs10401969	SUGP1/CILP2	intron	19	C	T	1.13	T2D	[62,85]
150	rs6017317	FITM2-R3HDML-HNF4A	intergenic	20	G	T	1.09	T2D	[63]
151	rs4812829	HNF4A	intron	20	A	G	1.09	T2D	[65]
152	rs5945326	DUSP9	intergenic	X	A	G	1.27	T2D	[25]
153	rs12010175	FAM58A	intron	X	G	A	1.21	T2D	[66]

List of common SNPs (Single Nucleotide Polymorphism) Associated with T2D (Type 2 Diabetes Mellitus), OR= Odd Ratio, RA= Risk Allele, OA= Odd Allele. Several loci have also reached evidence for association with HbA1c in type 1 and type 2diabetes, as well as in non-diabetic subjects, including loci near FN3K, HFE, TMPRSS6, ANK1, SPTA1, ATP11A/TUBGCP3, HK1, MTNR1B, GCK, G6PC2/ABCB11, TCF7L2, SLC30A8, SORCS1,

WDR72, GCS and BNC2 [204-207]. The associations with HbA1c may well in part be a function of hyperglycemia associated with five of the loci (TCF7L2, SLC30A8, GCK, G6PC2 and MTNR1B) [240,242,262-266]. Most of the others have been classified as novel, but some variants map to lociwhere more rare variants cause various forms of hereditary anemia and iron storage disorders. Common variants at these loci likely influence HbA1c levels via erythrocyte biology. Seven non-glycemic loci have shown to account for a 0.19 (% HbA1c) difference between the extreme 10% tails of the risk score,and would reclassify approximately 2% of a general white population screened for diabetes with HbA1c [267].

Genome Wide Association Study (GWAS)

Development of new genotyping technologies and the realization that we inherit stretches of the genometogether as haplotypes facilitated the cataloguing of common variants (HAPMAP, 1000 genomes) and allowed for new possibilities to apply unbiased global approaches to screen millions of common variantsfor association with complex diseases.[268,269]. *GWAs (Genome Wide Association) do not inevitably lead to identification of a gene or genes in a given locus associated with disease. Since the most strongly associated single nucleotide polymorphisms (SNPs) are often only markers for the functional variants responsible for the observed genetic effect and most associated regions harbour severalgenes, additional fine mapping of the loci in even larger sample sets is often necessary.[270].* Driven by the limitations of advances in genotyping technology, genome wide association scans (GWAS) have a generated a great deal of optimism among researchers working to identify susceptibility genes for Diabetes associated with nephropathy, neuropathy and retinopathy. The GWAs approach involves rapid scanning of many genetic markers (usually SNP's) in DNA samples from multiple individuals to detect common (minor allele frequency) genetic variation associated with diabetes mellitus. There are various studies reported uptill now relating search for genetic variations in Diabetes mellitus and correlating with patients having diabetes suffering with retinopathy, neuropathy, and nephropathy Table No (03).

Table 3. Showing common and uncommon genes name and class involved in Diabetes Nephropathy (DN), Diabetes Neuropathy (DNe), Diabetes Retinopathy (DR), Prediabetic Subject, Diabetic Subject.

Sr.No	Class	Gene name	Gene Code DNephr	Gene Code DNeuro	Gene Code DRetino	Gene code prediabetic	Gene code diabetic	Chromosome Location
1	Renin- angiotensin aldosterone System (RAAS)	Angiotensin converting Enzyme-1	ACE1	ACE1	-	-	-	17q23
		Angiotensinogen	AGT	-	-	AGT	AGT	1q42-43
		Angiotensin II Receptor	AGTR1	-		AGTR1	AGTR1	3q21-25
2	Glucose metabolism	Aldose Reductase	AKR1B	AKR1B	AKR1B1	AGTR1	AGTR1	17q35
		Glucose Transporter-1	SCL2A1	-	-	-	-	1p35
		Receptor for advanced glycosylation end products	RAGE	-	RAGE	-		6p21.3
3	Growth Factor	Transforming Growth factor Beta 1	TGFB1	-	TNFB1	TGFB1	TGFB1	19q13.1
		Transforming growth factor Beta Receptor I-III	TGFBR1/2/3	-	-	TGFBR1/2/3	TGFBR1/2/3	9q22, 3p22, 1p33
		Vascular endothelial	VEGF	VEGF	VEGF	VEGF	VEGF	6p12
		growth factor						
4	Oxidative Stress	Superoxide dismutase 1 & 2	SOD 1 / 2	-	-			21q22, 6p25.3
		Haptoglobin	HP	-	-			16q22
		Paroxonase	PON 1 / 2		-			7q21-22

#	Category	Gene	Symbol					Location
		Catalase	CAT	-	-	CAT	CAT	11p13
		Glutathione Peroxidase 1	GPX 1	-	-			3p21.3
5	Lipid Metabolism	Apolipoprotein E	APO E	APO E	-	APO E	APO E	19q13.2
		Adiponectin	ADIPOQ	-	-			3q27
		Peroxisome Proliferator activated receptor gamma	PPARG	-	-	PPARG	PPARG	3p25
		Apolipoprotein C-1	APO C1	-	-			19q13.2
6	Cytoskeletal Genes	Caldesmon	CALD	-	-			7q35
		B-assucin	ADD2	-	-			2p14
7	Inflammation	Intercellular Adhesion molecule-1	ICAM 1	-	ICAM1			19p13.3
		Interleukin-1	IL1B	IL-4, IL-10	-			2q14
8	Others	Endothelial nitric oxide synthase	NOS3	NOS3	-			7q36
		Protein Kinase C B1	PKCB1	-	PKCB1		PKCB1	16p11.0
		Erythropoetin	EPO	-	EPO			7q22
		Heparan Sulfate Proteoglycan 2	HEALTHYPG 2	-	-			1p36.1-p34
		FERM domain containing 3	FRMD3	-	-			9q21.32
		Cysteinyl tRNA synthetase	CARS	-	-			11p15.5

Chimerin 2	CHN2	-	-	7p15.3
Unc-13 homolog B	UNC13B	-	-	9p13.3
Gremin 1	GREM1	-	-	15q13.3
Carboxypetidase, Vitellogenic -like	CPVL	-	-	7p15.1
Alpha 2B Adrenergic receptor	-	Alpha 2B-IDR	-	
InterferonY	-	IFN-Y	-	
Emthylene tetra hydrofolate reductase	-	MTHFR	-	
Neuronal nitric oxide syntahase	-	NOS 1AP	-	
Toll like receptor-4	-	TLR4	-	
Pigment disorder reticulate	-	-	PDR	
High Temperature Requirement A Serine Peptidase 1	-	-	HTRA1	

Several common and uncommon genes and their class have been associated with diabetes and nephropathy (DN), neuropathy (DNe), and retinopathy (DR). This table lists the publications to identify a significant association of common variant genes related to diabetes and DN, DNe, and DR.

Largest GWAs to date, a multi stage approach that included African- American individuals with and without T2DM identified. several novel regions with evidence associated to T2D associated with Nephropathy, neuropathy, Retinopathy have been reported.[271-282] Although GWAs have identified several novel genes as potential contributors to DN, the approach is not without limitations. GWAs can be cofounded by population admixtures (combining multiple races for analysis) resulting in association due to differences between genetically distinct population. In addition GWAs to date have only evaluated common genetic variation using arrays which are not as comprehensive in their coverage of non European populations. While progress is being made with recent technological advances in GWAs objectively, genetic variants have not been identified that unambiguously define Diabetic Nephropathy, neuropathy and Retinopathy.

The most recent diabetes intermediary trait assessed by a GWA scan was proinsulin level. Proinsulin is a precursor of mature insulin and C-peptide. Higher circulating proinsulin levels are associated with impaired ü-cell function, raised glucose levels, insulin resistance, and type 2 diabetes [283]. Nine SNPs at eight loci have shown association with proinsulin levels [284]. Two loci (*LARP6* and *SGSM2*) have not been previously related to metabolic traits, one (*MADD*) has been associated with fasting glucose, one (*PCSK1*) has been implicated in obesity, and four (*TCF7L2, SLC30A8, VPS13C/C2CD4A/B*, and *ARAP1*, formerly *CENTD2*) increase type 2 diabetes risk. The proinsulin- raising allele of *ARAP1* was associated with a lower fasting glucose, improved ü-cell function and lower risk of type 2 diabetes. There is no doubt that genetic studies on glycemic traits have and will continue to illuminate the biology underlying glucose homeostasis and type 2 diabetes development.

CHAPTER IV- MATERIALS AND METHODS

Study Design

This a genome wide association, observational cross sectional study analyzing the gene expression level and there correlation with metabolic pathways in diabetic, prediabetic compared with healthy control.

For this study we have used blood samples from Diabetic, Prediabetic and Healthy subjects from MGM medical college and Hospital, Aurangabad. Data obtained from subjects have been analysed for Differential Expression of Genes (DEG) and Gene Ontology (GO).

Research Question

"Which are the genes responsible for the diabetic and prediabetic stage, compared with healthy subject, how those gene effect the gene ontology, different pathways. If there are some differential gene found is they can be targeted to normalize the diabetic, prediabetic status."

Selection of study subjects

The subjects included in our research work were short listed from the Medicine Dept, in MGM Hospitaland College, Aurangabad. Subjects for the study were recruited from the hospital staff, Teacher and patients.

The study population for the present study was divided into three groups as follows:-

Group I:- healthy subject as control for comparison were included in this group

Group II:- Patient with pre Diabetic who on clinical evaluation (HBA1C)

Group III:- Patient with diabetic who on clinical evaluation (HBA1C)

All the subjects of our study were enrolled and assigned to one of the above three group afterverifying their compliance with the following inclusion and exclusion criteria. In order to ensure the closest possible match between the three groups, 3 individual were selected based oninclusion and exclusion criteria.

Inclusion and exclusion Criteria

> ➤ Inclusion Criteria:

All the subjects were enrolled and categorised based on ADA 2016 Criteria.

Table 4. Parameters for Diabetic and Prediabetic subject

Diagnosis	Gender	Age (years)	Fasting plasma glucose	2-hour OGTT	HbA1C
Normal (Healthy)	Male	55	<100mg/dl (%.6 mmol/l)	<140 mg/dl (7.8 mmol/l)	<5.7 %
Pre-Diabetes	Male	72	100-125 mg/dl (5.6-6.9 mmol/l)	140-199 mg/dl (7.8-11.0 mmol/l)	5.7-6.4%
Diabetes	Male	68	$\geq$126 mg/dl (7.0 mmol/l)	$\geq$ 200 mg/dl (11.1 mmol/l	$\geq$ 6.5%

Table showing Range of Diabetic and prediabetic by American Diabetic Association (ADA) 2016 (1)

> ➤ Exclusion Criteria:-

- Subject who denied consent to be a part of the study.
- Previous illnesses of any systematic / infective/ toxic/ genetic/ metabolic disorders.
- Alcoholic subjects.
- Subjects consuming medications- Steroids, Protease inhibitors, antipsychotics, diuretics,vitamins as they affect glucose homeostasis.

Clinical Assessment

All the subjects under the study were evaluated clinically by physicians at the MGM Medical College and Hospital, Aurangabad. A complete lipid profile and HBA1C and Questionnaire were completed to obtain demographic data, medical history including drugs, and lifestyle factors.

Collection of Blood Sample and Analysis

Blood samples were obtained after an overnight fast. Under all aseptic precautions a single sample of venous blood was obtained from all participants. The obtained sample were sent to the central laboratoryand analysed for FPG, HBA1C, total Cholesterol and triglycerides.

Once haematological result obtained blood sample has been transported Xcelris Lab Ltd, Ahmedabad approved by MGM University of Health Sciences, Aurangabad for the purpose of Whole Transcriptome Analysis (WTA).

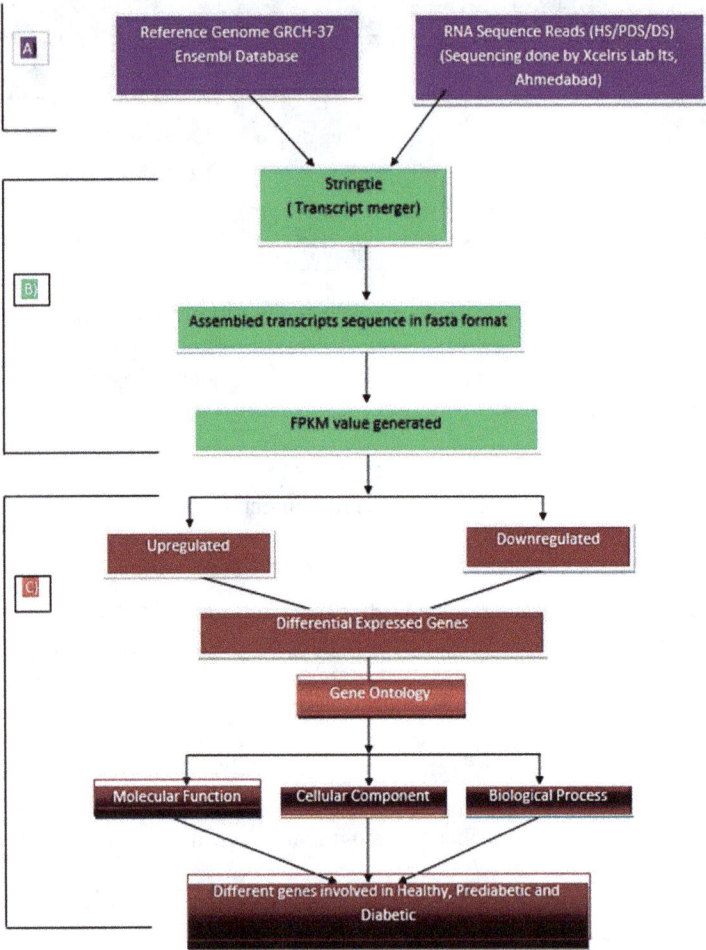

Flow Diagram of Transciptomic Analysis (NGS) of healthy, prediabetic and diabetic subject, Study has been differentiated into 3 segments :-

A) Reference genome GrCh 37.p13 downloaded from ensembl, and Blood sample extracted from subjects has been sent to sequencing outsourced by Xcelris Lab Ltd, Ahmedabad.

B) Transcirpt merge between samples and reference genome GrCh 37.p13 and assembled them with fasta file format and generate FPKM Value

C) Generated FPKM value has been used to obtain Differentially Expressed Genes (DEG) and GeneOntology (GO) in Healthy, prediabetic and Diabetic sample.

Analysis process of the samples in the Lab

In Xcleris Lab ltd, Ahmedabad where isolation, qualitative and quantitative analysis of RNA was isolated from samples diabetic, prediabetic and healthy by Trizol method (296). Total qualtiy of RNA was checked by 1% formaldehyde, denaturing agarose gel and quantified using Nanodrop 8000 spectrophotometer. Library preparation were prepared using Illumina Truseq RNA kit v2, briefly double stranded cDNA was subjected to end repair of overhangs resulting from fragmentation. The end repaired fragments were A-tailed,adapter ligated and then enriched by limited number of PCR cycles. The amplified libraries were analysed on Bioanalyzer 2100 (agilent technologies). After obtaining the Qubit Concetration for the library and the mean peak size from bioanalyzer profile, libraries were loaded into illumina platform for cluster generation and sequencing. Paired end sequencing allows the template fragments to be sequenced in both the forward and reverse directions. The library molecule binds to complementary adapter oligos on paired end flow cell. The adapter were designed to allow selective cleavage of the forward strands after resynthesis of the reverse strand during sequencing. The copied reverse strand was then used to sequence from the opposite end of the fragments.

Bioinformatics Data mining and analysis

further Bioinformatics study has been processed for mapping reads, transcript assembly, Differential Gene Expression, Pathway Analysis and there inferential, descriptive statistics is undertaken of said subjects Healthy, Prediabetic and Diabetic.

Data normalisation is applied to remove systematic biases in the data. The goal of inferential statistics is undertaken to evaluate gene expression changes in term of significance and confidence.

Log Intensity- Differential expression analysis primary objective here to access the mRNA transcripts level the appropriate statistical technique applied using log intensity value of gene expression, Variate, multivariate distribution, Normal probability Plot, Correlation coefficient of all 3 subjects.

The approach provides the fold change value considering the scatter of observation and their by provides Up and Down regulated genes across the sample.

The reference genome of Human (GRch37.p13, genome Size 3.2 Gb) and the corresponding GTF file was downloaded from Ensembl database (reference GTF contain 332743047 bp).

Mapping HQ Reads:- Mapping of all the read of all 3 samples done against the Homo Sapiens (GrCh37.p13) to identify the positions from where the reads originated. **HISAT** (Hierarchical indexing for spliced alignment of transcripts) and **String tie** are free open source software's, tool for comprehensive analysis of RNA-sequence. Together these software's allow aligning reads to a genome, assembling transcripts including novel splice variants, and computing the abundance of each sample and compare to identify Differential Expressed Genes (DEG) and transcripts.

This mapping information allows us to collect subset of the reads corresponds to each gene and then they are assembled and quantification of transcripts done which represents by those reads.

Transcript assembly: - Transcript assembly has been developed using String Tie program , which tries to assemble all the reaDiabetic in the group into distinct gene loci and then assembling each locus into asmany isoforms as needed to explain. String Tie simultaneously assembles and quantify the final transcripts. The GTF (Gene Transfer Format) annotation files, containing exon-intron structures of "known" genes, are then used to annotate the assembled transcripts and quantify the expression of known genes which gave a clue to novel transcript found in Healthy, prediabetic and diabetic subjects. The output consists of assembled gene/transcript GTF file for all the 3 samples, which produced3,17,407 transcripts.

Differential Expression Analysis: differential gene expression was performed of 3 different samples of different subjects, abundance of merged transcripts in all the samples were estimated using String-Tie in the form of FPKM (fragments per kilobase per million reads mapped) using the formula:-

82

$$FPKM = \frac{\text{number of reads of the region} \ X \ 10^9 \text{Length of}}{\text{transcript} \ X \ \text{Total number of reads mapped}}$$

$$Log2FC = Log\ 2\ (B) - Log\ 2\ (A)$$

The log 2 transformed fold change values was analyzed for deciding the genes for up-regulated and down-regulated, criteria used to identify up-regulated and down-regulated genes along with the significance is log2FC>0 will be considered for up-regulated, log2FC<0 is considered for down- regulated. Top 50 significantly expressed genes (highly up and down regulated genes).

Pathway Analysis: - Ortholog assignment and mapping of the transcripts to the biological pathways were performed using KEGG automatic annotation server (KAAS). All the differentially expressed genes were compared against the KEGG database using BLASTX with bit score value of 60 (default). The mapped transcripts represent metabolic pathways of major Biomolecules such as carbohydrates, lipids, nucleotides, amino acids, glycans. The mapped genes also represent the genes involved in metabolism, genetic information their processes, environmental information their processes and cellular process. (Metabolism, genetic information processing, environmental information processing, cellular processes, organismal system, human diseases).

Gene ontology (GO):-, can be studied to know the involvement of genes is towards, Upregulated or Downregulated, GO provides controlled vocabulary of defined terms representing gene products and there properties like Cellular Component, Biological Process, Molecular function. In gene ontology information regarding part of cells or its extracellular environment can be studied, also some elemental activities of a gene product at molecular level can be highlighted, also operations or sets of molecular events with defined beginning and end.

Qualitative Model Energy Analysis (Q-MEAN):- Q-Mean Z score indicates the quality score of the model and provides the structural validation where implementing this score clear structural differences can be visualize also fluctuations in the score can be documented in the subjects. QMEAN and agreement terms range from 0 to 1 and the statistical potential terms deliver pseudo energies with negative values for energetically favourable states. In the Z-score calculations, we adjusted the sign of the statistical terms such that higher Z-score consistently relate to favourable states, i.e. higher QMEAN Z-score means better agreement with predicted features and lower mean force potential energy.

Statistical Analysis

All the sequence data obtained was collected in BAM, GTT file format which was opened in Notepad++ Application, then they are processed further and opened into excel sheet, which further wascompiled and statistical analysis performed using SPSS version 24.0[th] . Normality of data was assessed by using Shapiro-Wilk test, in given below table shapiro-wilk test all the variables found to be significant , all variable data was not normally distributed (table 5). So for analysis of this data non- parametric test was applied.

Table 5. Normality test by Shapiro-Wilk test

	Shapiro-Wilk Test		
	Statistic	df	Sig.
FPKM_HEALTHY UR	0.726	25	P=0.000 S
FPKM_PREDIABETIC UR	0.788	25	P=0.0001 S
FPKM DIABETIC UR	0.596	25	P<0.0001 S
FPKM_HEALTHY DR	0.908	25	P=0.027 S
FPKM_PREDIABETIC DR	0.749	25	P<0.0001 S
FPKM DIABETIC DR	0.823	25	P=0.001 S

*UR=Up regulated, DR=Downregulated

Mean and SD (Standard Deviation) were calculated for quantitative variables and proportions were calcuated for categorical variables. Also data was represented in form of visual impression like Histogram, Bar Diagram, venn diagram, heat map etc. For comparison of Up and Down regulation in different groups Kruskal Wallis Test was applied (table 6 & 7). For comparison of mean difference between two groups Mann Whitney test was applied. Also F-value, T-test was used to check significant difference between groups. Chi-Square test was applied to check significant differences between two attributes. P-value <0.05 was considered statistically significant.

84

Table 6. Comparison of Mean TOP 25 for Upregulated [Kruskal-Wallis test.]

Samples	N	Mean±SD	95% CI		Chi- Square value	P-value
			Lower	Upper		
FPKM_HEALTHY UR	25	0.01661380±0.022317067	0.0074017 7	0.02582583		
FPKM_PREDIABE TIC UR	25	0.93402956±0.927404338	0.5512158 6	1.31684326	47.49	**P<0.0001S**
FPKM DIABETIC UR	25	0.62745716±0.876880380	0.2654987 3	0.98941559		

*UR=Upregulation

Mean & S.D value of healthy (0.0166), prediabetic (0.9340) and diabetic (0.6274) up regulated is observed based on Kruskal wallis test the mean found significant in all studied subjects, also Chi-squaretest is 47.49 observed in UP Regulation.

Table 7. Comparison of Mean TOP 25 for Downregulated [Kruskal-Wallis test.]

Samples	N	Mean±SD	95% CI		Chi-Square value	P-value
			Lower	Upper		
FPKM_HEALTH DR	25	0.56180320±0.347047164	0.41854917	0.70505723	41.43	**P<0.0001 S**
FPKM_PREDIA BETIC DR	25	0.02581628±0.088449777	-0.01069399	0.06232655		
FPKM DIABETIC DR	25	0.00717148±0.006406731	0.00452691	0.00981605		

*DR= Down regulation

Mean and S.D Value of healthy (0.5618), prediabetic (0.2581), diabetic= (0.0071) is DOWN regulated is observed based on Kruskal Wallis Test the values found to be significant in all subjects, also chi- square test is 41.43 is observed in DOWN Regulation.

Terminologies

a) Transcripts:- it can be defined as step of gene expression, in which a particular segment of DNA is copied to RNA (especially m rNA) which codes for protein with the help of enzyme RNA Polymerase.

b) Reads:- it is an inferred sequence of base pairs (or base pair probabilities) corresponding to all or part of single DNA fragment. Typical sequencing experiment involves fragmentation of the genome into millions of molecules, which are size-selected and ligated to adapters.
c) UP and DOWN Regulation:- In Biological context of eukaryotic and prokaryotic organisms production of gene products, DOWN- Regulation is the process by which a cell decreases the quantity of cellular components, such as protein, ontology, and enzymes produced for metabolic pathways, in response to external stimulus, the complementary process that involves increase ofsuch components is called upregulation.

Ethical Approval

The study was approved by the ethical committee of MGM Institute of Health Sciences, Aurangabad(MGM-ECRHS/2014/233) and informed consents for the studies was taken from all the subjects.

Chapter V. Results

Figure 7. Quality Check of total RNA run on 1% Formaldehyde Agarose Gel

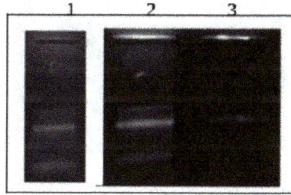

Figure shows the quality by 1% formaldehyde agarose gel electrophoresis of small and large subunit and purity of the sample lane 1 healthy, lane 2 diabetic, and lane 3 prediabetic where we can observe 28s (large subunit), 18s (small subunit) and 5s (large subunit) Svedberg unit, where some over expression can be observed in lane 2 and lane 3.

Table 8. Quantification using NanoDrop 8000 Spectrophotometer:

LaneNo	Sample ID	Concentration (ng/µl)	Yield (µg)	A260/280
1	Healthy	278	5.5	2.01
2	Diabetic	326	6.5	1.97
3	Prediabetic	242	4.8	1.89

Quantification and concentration of Healthy, Prediabetic and Diabetic subject using Nanodrop 8000 Spectrophotometer, as compared with standard ratio given (ammyyappan etal 2009) for macromolecules, where purity of RNA is 2.0, in Healthy Subject it has been observed 2.0, whereas in Prediabetic it is 1.89 and in Diabetic 1.97 has been observed.

Table 9. Standard Ratio of Macromolecules by Ammyyappan et al 2009

Purity of	Target A260/280 Ratio
DNA	1.8
RNA	2.0
Protein	0.6

Figure 8. Bioanalyzer profiles of Heathy, prediabetic and Diabetic libraries on Agilent Chip

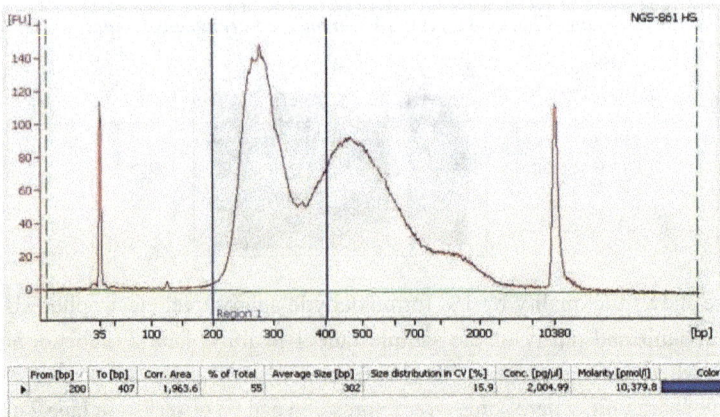

From [bp]	To [bp]	Corr. Area	% of Total	Average Size [bp]	Size distribution in CV [%]	Conc. [pg/µl]	Molarity [pmol/l]	Color
200	407	1,963.6	55	302	15.9	2,004.99	10,379.8	

Sows the mRNA Library profile of sample Healthy Subject, PreDiabetic Subject and Diabetic Subjecton Agilent DNA Chip the mean size of the libraries were 302 bp the library were sequenced using 2 X150 bp pair end on Illumina Platform.

Figure 9. Statistics of high quality sequencing data

File Name	Total Reads (Forward+Reverse)	Total Bases
Diabetic_forward	58,588,906	8,233,839,132
Diabetic_reverse		
Healthy_ forward	56,578,880	7,842,978,223
Healthy_reverse		
Prediabetic_forward	52,857,644	7,391,654,813
Prediabetic_reverse		

Shows the High quality sequence data has been generated based on forward and reverse operon model, total bases and total reads found at both the end by 2 X 150 bp on Illumina Platform of Healthy, Prediabetic and Diabetic Samples.

Sample name	Total reads	Total mapped reads
Healthy	56578880	42711396
Prediabetic	52857644	40816672
Diabetic	58588906	54534553

Showing total number of transcript reads founds in Healthy Subject, Prediabetic Subject and Diabetic Subject and mapped with Reference Genome GrCh37.p13. with Healthy, prediabetic and Diabetic

Graph 1. Mapped reads with Reference genome GrCh37.p13

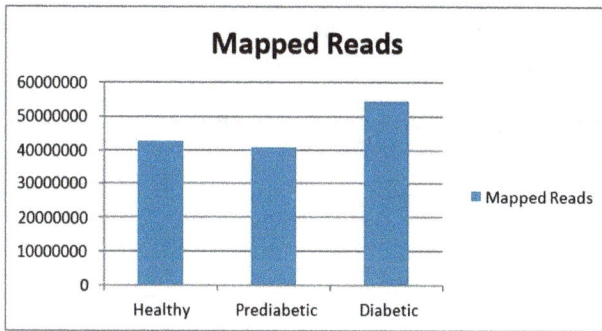

Shows the Graphical representing of numbers of reads mapped on RNA library in Healthy, Prediabetic and Diabetic Subject where Diabetic subject shows more mapped reads as compared to Healthy and Prediabetic Sample.

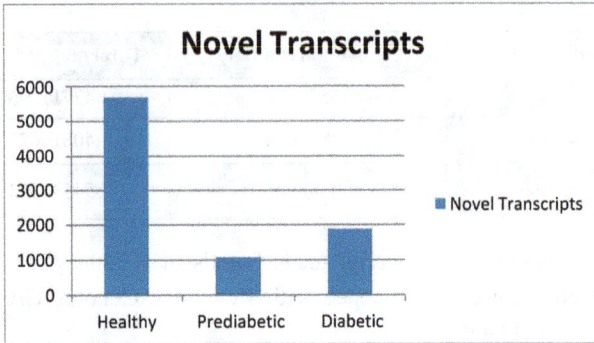

Graphically represents the number of novel transcripts found on Healthy, Prediabetic and Diabetic subject, where as compared to Healthy Prediabetic and diabetic have less number of novel transcripts, where Healthy shows 5684 number of novel genes in transcript library, where in Prediabetic 1085, and diabetic 1890 genes are observed.

Table 11. Description of genomics elements obtained from Reference Genome of Human (GrCh37.p13genome Size 3.2 Gb)

Total base pairs in the genome	3326743047
Coding genes	20805
Pseudogenes	14181
Gene transcripts	196501

Shows the genomic elements :- Coding genes, Pseudogenes, Gene Transcripts and total base pairs inReference Genome GrCh37.p13, downloaded from Ensembl Database in GTF format.

Table 12. Mapping statistics of Healthy, Prediabetic and Diabetic Samples with Reference Genome (GrCh 37.p13).

Sample name	Total reads	Total mapped reads
healthy	56578880	5579960218
prediabetic	52857644	6056347784
diabetic	58588906	7664057464

Shows the statistics of healthy. Prediabetic and diabetic samples where there libraries have been individually mapped with reference genome (GrCh37.p13) using HISAT (hierarchical indexing for spliced alignment of transcripts) Builder has been used to obtained the total mapped reads.

Table 13. Statistics of only transcript which has been assembled in Healthy, prediabetic and diabetic sample with individual mapped with Reference Genome (GrCh37.p13)

samplename	Total transcript	Total length of all transcripts (bp)	Maximum Length (bp)
Healthy	176186	85944929	91667
Prediabetic	140088	58889958	91667
Diabetic	34526	31111062	91667

Shows the transcripts which has been assembled with reference genome and individual with Healthy, prediabetic and diabetic samples where approximately 91667 length of Base pairs have been obtained in all studied samples, where as total transcripts values in all samples have been found in differentnumbers.

Graph 3. Gene Transcripts found in Healthy, Prediabetic and Diabetic samples individually mapped with Reference Genome GrCh37.p13.

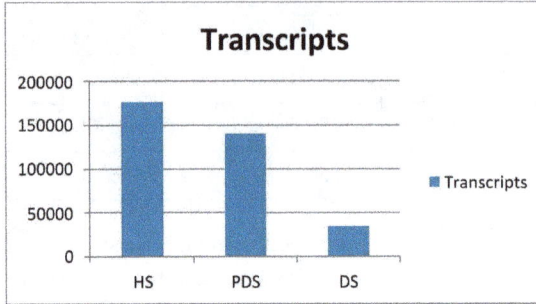

*HS=Healthy, PDS=Prediabetic, DS=Diabetic

Graphically representing the number of transcripts variants observed in Healthy, prediabetic and Diabetic samples individually mapped with Reference Genome (GrCh37.p13) where genetic fluctuations have been observed i.e very less number in Diabetic 34526 genes, as compare with healthy and prediabetic.

Differential Expression Analysis

Abundances of the merged transcripts in all the samples were estimated using StringTie in the form ofFPKM (fragments per kilobase per million reads mapped) values. The formula is provided below:

Figure 10. Implemented formula to calculate the FPKM (fragments per kilobase per million reaDiabeticmapped) Value

$$FPKM= \frac{\text{number of reads of the region} \times 10^9}{\text{Length of transcript} \times \text{total number of reads mapped}}$$

Shows the formula used to calculate the FPKM (fragments per kilobase per million reads mapped) value of each reads obtained from library and with the reference genome GrCh37.p13, where number of reaDiabetic obtained divide by length of transcripts obtained from healthy, prediabetic and diabetic sample multiplied by number of reads mapped with studied sample and Reference Genome GrCh37.p13.

Figure 11. Log 2 Transform value Formula

$$\text{Log2FC} = \text{Log 2 (B)} - \text{Log 2 (A)}$$

Showing formula for Log2FC normalization used for measure describing the quantity changes betweenoriginal and subsequent measurements, defined as ratio between two quantities A and B, then fold change of B with respect to A is B/A [296].

Table 14. Log 2 Transformed fold change value parameter used to decide Upregulated and Downregulated genes in Healthy, Prediabetic and Diabetic sample

Key	Status
Log2FC > 0	Upregulated
Log2FC < 0	Down regulated

Table No:14 showing the LOG 2 Transformed fold change value used to bifurcate the up-regulation anddown-regulation process of genes based on there FPKM Value, if observed value is more than zero is counted in up-regulation stream vice versa log 2Fc value is less than or Zero is considered

Table 15. Statistics of differentially expressed genes (DEG) expressed in Healthy vs Prediabetic and Diabetic

Samples	Exclusively expressed in Controlsample	Exclusively expressed in Treated sample	Upregulated	Downregulated
healthy_vs_diabetic	6091	946	496	1809
healthy_vs_prediabetic	4853	1992	1596	1947

Showing the stastistics of control sample (Healthy), Treated (Prediabetic and Diabetic samples) and their differential Expressed Genes (DEG) and there distribution in up and down regulation process in cell regulations, where in control vs treated i.e Healthy vs diabetic more numbers of genes were observed in down-regulation as it would have to be in up-regulation, where as in healthy vs Prediabetic some slight fluctuations has been observed in up and down regulation process.

Figure 12. Heat map of highly significant differential expressed genes in Healthy, Prediabetic and Diabetic samples

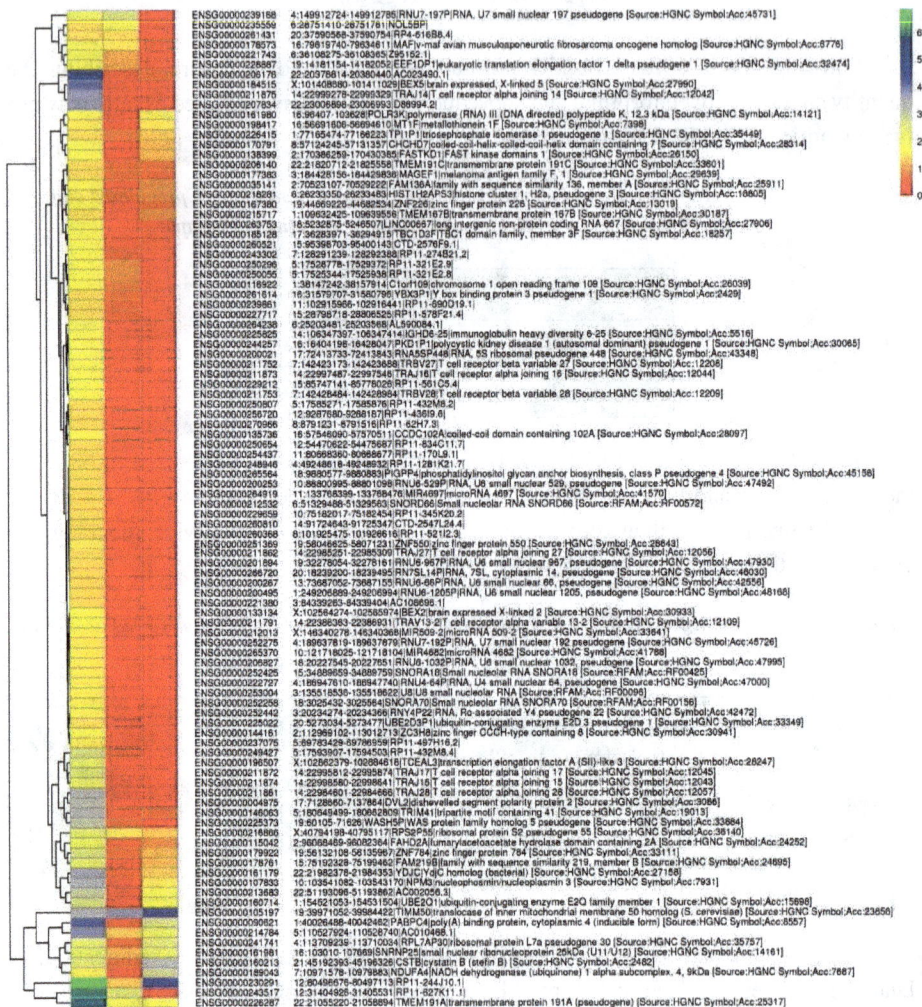

Heatmap representing top 50 up-regulated (25) and down-regulated (25) genes was plotted using FPKM values for Healthy, Prediabetic and Diabetic sample comparison. The color coding ranges from red to green where shades of red represent lowly expressed genes and shades of green represents highly expressed genes. Where most of the genes are represented in Red in prediabetic and diabetic samples which concludes the low level expression of genes in said sample, as compared to healthy Green and Yellow are observed in healthy sample which indicates the high and intermediate level of expression are observed.

Table 16. List of top 50 genes shortlisted based on FPKM value on up and down regulated in healthy, prediabetic and diabetic samples

GeneID	Description	FPKM_Healthy	FPKM_Prediabetic	FPKM_Diabetic
ENSG00000230291	12:80496676-80497113|RP11-244J10.1|	6.87571	1.27116	4.3959
ENSG00000243517	12:31404926-31405531|RP11-627K11.1|	5.988127	2.59954	0.3506
ENSG00000226287	22:21055220-21058894|TMEM191A|	5.886	1.73292	1.7622
ENSG00000206176	22:20378814-20380440|AC023490.1|	4.624961	0	0.5785
ENSG00000090621	1:40026488-40042462|PABPC4|	4.171378	0.50003	2.6754
ENSG00000184515	X:101408680-101411029|BEX5|	4.093974	0	0
ENSG00000214784	5:110527924-110528740|AC010468.1|	3.842479	1.36423	2.2657
ENSG00000211875	14:22999278-22999329|TRAJ14|	3.759193	0	0
ENSG00000207834	22:23006898-23006993|D86994.2|	3.758778	0	0
ENSG00000161179	22:21982378-21984353|YDJC|	3.579013	0.47664	1.3199
ENSG00000107833	10:103541082-103543170|NPM3|	3.472191	0.3016	1.5278
ENSG00000105197	19:39971052-39984422|TIMM50|	3.43851	3.72519	4.2811
ENSG00000146063	5:180649499-180662809|TRIM41|	3.371217	0.39628	0.6658
ENSG00000211861	14:22984601-22984666|TRAJ28|	3.351187	0.11221	0
ENSG00000004975	17:7128660-7137864|DVL2|	3.292973	0.35936	0.1746
ENSG00000225373	19:60105-71626|WASH5P|	3.117771	0.62513	0.3403
ENSG00000213683	22:51193096-51193862|AC002056.3|	3.091671	0.35332	1.7987
ENSG00000179922	19:56132108-56135967|ZNF784|	2.743139	0.66745	1.1607
ENSG00000160714	1:154521053-154531504|UBE2Q1|	2.661996	0	1.9461
ENSG00000249427	5:17593907-17594503|RP11-432M8.4|	2.635856	0.55447	0.0222
ENSG00000160213	21:45192393-45196326|CSTB|	2.522228	0.62088	3.3501
ENSG00000211872	14:22995812-22995874|TRAJ17|	2.521819	0	0
ENSG00000178761	15:75192328-75199462|FAM219B|	2.479663	0.4348	1.2366
ENSG00000241741	4:113709239-113710034|RPL7AP30|	2.422217	0.66055	2.6306
ENSG00000216866	X:40794198-40795117|RPS2P55|	2.39568	1.52807	1.2677
ENSG00000196507	X:102862379-102884618|TCEAL3|	2.35505	0.1222	0.287

Gene ID	Locus	Gene		
ENSG00000161981	16:103010-107669|SNRNP25|	2.340191	1.22212	2.2975
ENSG00000211874	14:22998580-22998641|TRAJ15|	2.25265	0	0
ENSG00000115042	2:96068469-96082364|FAHD2A|	2.156621	0.46637	0.9045
ENSG00000239168	4:149912724-149912785|	2.076792	2.74282	0
ENSG00000264238	6:25203481-25203568|AL590084.1|	1.935193	0	0
ENSG00000170791	8:57124245-57131357|CHCHD7|	1.883084	0.28956	1.2074
ENSG00000250296	5:17528778-17529372|RP11-321E2.9|	1.875665	0.8039	0.0533
ENSG00000178573	16:79619740-79634611|MAF|	1.825737	1.59259	0.3834
ENSG00000225825	14:106347397-106347414|GHD6-25|	1.817193	0	0
ENSG00000185128	17:36283971-36294915|TBC1D3F|	1.802164	0.31976	0.3474
ENSG00000260521	15:95398703-95400143|CTD-2576F9.1|	1.770083	0.4417	0.4053
ENSG00000229212	15:85747141-85778026|RP11-561C5.4|	1.766247	0.13961	0.1548
ENSG00000243302	7:128291239-128292388|RP11-274B21.2|	1.748117	0.54341	0.0551
ENSG00000211753	7:142428484-142428984|TRBV28|	1.744448	0	0.1474
ENSG00000200021	17:72413733-72413843|RNA5SP448|	1.740015	0	0
ENSG00000221743	6:36108275-36108365|Z95152.1|	1.734464	1.09713	0
ENSG00000211752	7:142423173-142423688|TRBV27|	1.734014	0	0
ENSG00000263753	18:5232875-5246507|LINC00667|	1.733856	0.1745	0.4354
ENSG00000211873	14:22997487-22997546|TRAJ16|	1.73066	0	0
ENSG00000250055	5:17525344-17525938|RP11-321E2.8|	1.720421	0.82607	0.0178
ENSG00000244257	16:16404198-16428047|PKD1P1|	1.704175	0	0
ENSG00000116922	1:38147242-38157914|C1orf109|	1.657401	0.72077	0.0247
ENSG00000133134	X:102564274-102565974|BEX2|	1.652201	0	0.0476
ENSG00000228887	19:14181154-14182052|EEF1DP1|	1.650074	1.03689	0.3903
ENSG00000161980	16:96407-103628|POLR3K|	1.642553	0.22443	1.9115
ENSG00000135736	16:57546090-57570511|CCDC102A|	1.634638	0.23787	0.1492
ENSG00000144161	2:112969102-113012713|ZC3H8|	1.63186	0.06462	0.2103
ENSG00000138399	2:170386259-170430385|FASTKD1|	1.630332	0.10737	1.1561
ENSG00000035141	2:70523107-70529222|FAM136A|	1.617689	0.30065	0.8986

Gene ID	Description			
ENSG00000167380	19:44669226-44682534|ZNF226|	1.617593	0	0.6413
ENSG00000211791	14:22386363-22386931|TRAV13-2|	1.610147	0	0
ENSG00000189043	7:10971578-10979883|NDUFA4|NADH dehydrogenase (ubiquinone) 1 alpha subcomplex, 4, 9kDa [Source:HGNC Symbol;Acc:7687]	1.590473	0.35464	2.9023
ENSG00000198417	16:56691606-56694610|MT1F|	1.580342	0.03557	1.5075
ENSG00000252275	4:189637819-189637879|RNU7-192P|	1.557594	0	0
ENSG00000265370	10:121718025-121718104|MIR4682|	1.557594	0	0
ENSG00000253004	3:135518536-135518622|U8|	1.536707	0	0
ENSG00000252258	18:3025432-3025564|SNORA70|	1.530268	0	0
ENSG00000237075	5:69783429-69786959|RP11-497H16.2|	1.529394	0.11425	0.1661
ENSG00000218281	6:26233350-26233483|HIST1H2APS3|	1.528535	0.62021	0.865
ENSG00000212013	X:146340278-146340368|MIR509-2|	1.523361	0	0.0582
ENSG00000206827	18:20227545-2027651|RNU6-1032P|	1.513923	0	0
ENSG00000252425	15:34489659-34489759|SNORA18|	1.511329	0	0
ENSG00000252442	3:20234274-20234366|RNY4P22|	1.51014	0	0.2316
ENSG00000222727	4:186947610-186947740|RNU4-64P|	1.510034	0	0
ENSG00000251369	19:58046625-58071231|ZNF550|	1.490938	0	0
ENSG00000256720	12:9287680-9288187|RP11-43619.6|	1.479408	0.19977	0
ENSG00000211862	14:22985251-22985309|TRAJ27|	1.478394	0	0
ENSG00000225022	20:5273034-5273447|UBE2D3P|ubiquitin conjugating enzyme E2D 3 pseudogene 1 [Source:HGNC Symbol;Acc:33349]	1.470476	0	0.1694
ENSG00000215717	1:109632425-109639556|TMEM167B|	1.465304	0.0854	0.8207
ENSG00000200267	13:73687052-73687155|RNU6-66P|	1.457748	0	0
ENSG00000200495	1:249206889-249206994|RNU6-1205P|	1.457183	0	0
ENSG00000221380	3:84339263-84339404|AC108696.1|	1.457045	0	0

ENSG00000260368	8:101925475-101926616|RP11-52I12.3|	1.453709	0.05428	0.0449
ENSG00000226415	1:77165474-77166223|TPI1P1|	1.453408	0.68973	1.2761
ENSG00000266720	20:18239200-18239495|RN7SL14P|	1.44972	0	0
ENSG00000250807	5:17585271-17585876|RP11-432M8.2|	1.445273	0.33351	0.011
ENSG00000239861	11:102915966-102916441|RP11-690D19.1|	1.444701	0.46098	0
ENSG00000201894	19:32278054-32278161|RNU6-967P|	1.425391		0
ENSG00000250654	12:54470622-54475687|RP11-834C11.7|	1.42527	0.21503	0.26
ENSG00000206140	22:21820712-21825558|TMEM191C|	1.423753	0.6297	0.6661
ENSG00000227717	15:28798718-28806525|RP11-578F21.4|	1.423111	0.56043	0
ENSG00000229659	10:75182017-75184254|RP11-345K20.2|	1.418904	0	0.0528
ENSG00000261614	16:31579707-31580796|YBX3P1|Y box binding protein 3 pseudogene 1	1.416601	0.65828	0.2782
ENSG00000235559	6:28751410-2875178|NOL5BP|	1.413838	1.90449	0
ENSG00000200253	10:88800995-88801098|RNU6-529P|	1.412817	0	0
ENSG00000264919	11:133768399-133768476|MIR4697|	1.407825	0	0
ENSG00000212532	6:51329488-51329563|SNORD66|	1.4073	0	0
ENSG00000177383	3:184428156-184429836|MAGEF1|	1.405788	0.63618	0.551
ENSG00000260810	14:91724643-91725347|CTD-2547L24.4|	1.40478	0	0.0727
ENSG00000248946	4:49248618-49248932|RP11-1281K21.7|	1.402451	0	0
ENSG00000270966	8:8791231-8791516|RP11-62H7.3|	1.402379	0.21674	0
ENSG00000261431	20:37590568-37590754|RP4-616B8.4|	1.402112	1.46528	0
ENSG00000265564	18:9880577-9880883|PIGPP4|	1.402004	0	0
ENSG00000254437	11:80668360-80668677|RP11-170L9.1|	1.391059	0	0
		210.8574	40.9926	55.81

Showing the common list of gene ID based on FPKM in all subject Healthy Subject, Prediabetic Subject and Diabetic Subject , with their chromosome location and Start and End point. In above table pink colorshows the NADH ubiquinine one of the important enzyme utilized in Oxidative phosphorylation (Electron Transport Chain) Q cycle, where different values of FPKM has been observed in Healthy, Prediabetic and Diabetic samples.

Table 17. Showing th number of genes expressed differentially in Healthy, prediabetic and diabetic sample

Exclusively Expressed in Healthy	4854
Exclusively expressed in Prediabetic	1993
Exclusively expressed in Diabetic	946

Graph 4. Bar Diagram showing the differentially expressed genes in healthy, prediabetic and diabetic

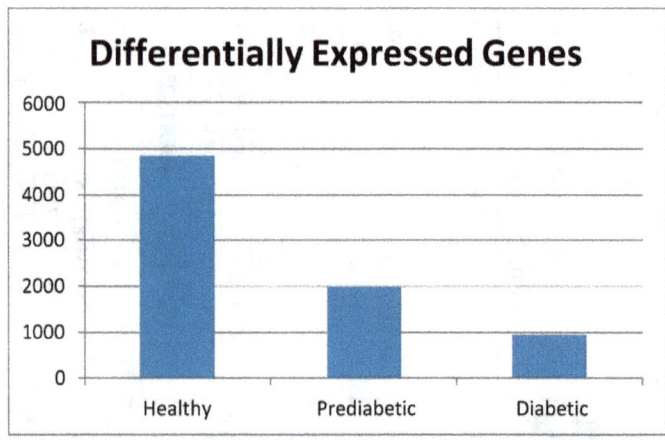

Shows the number of genes exclusively expressed in studied samples (Healthy, prediabetic and Diabetic) and graphically they have plotted to show the variation and fluctuation between the samples.

Table 18. Showing the numbers of Genes differentially expressed in healthy and prediabetic and variations in UP and Down Regulation

Healthy vs Prediabetic	
DGE	3544
Up	1597
Down	1948

Graph 5. Bar Graph showing the numbers of Genes differentially expressed in healthy and prediabeticand variations in UP and Down Regulation

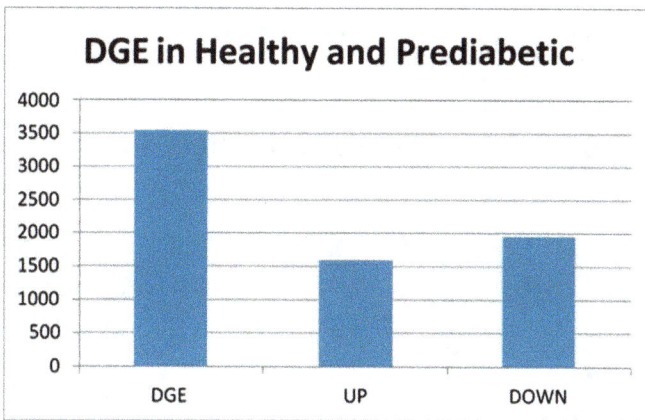

*DGE= Differential Gene Expression, UP=Upregulation, DR=Downregulation

Showing the numbers of genes differentially expressed in healthy vs prediabetic based on their FPKM value, graphical representation shows the variation in UP and DOWN regulation stream, more numberof genes are observed in Down regulation and comparatively less number in UP regulation are observed.

Table 19. Showing the numbers of genes differentially expressed in healthy and diabetic and variationsin up and down regulation

Healthy vs Diabetic	
DGE	2306
UP	497
DOWN	1810

*DGE= Differential Gene Expression, UP=Upregulation, DR=Downregulation

Graph 6. Showing the numbers of genes differentially expressed in healthy and diabetic and variations inup and down regulation of cell regulation

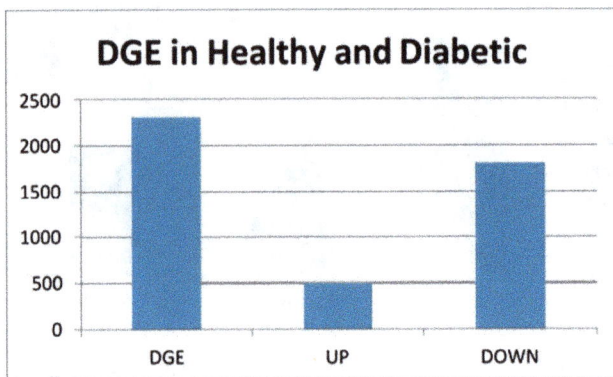

DGE in Healthy and Diabetic

*DGE= Differential Gene Expression, UP=Upregulation, DR=Downregulation

Showing the numbers of genes differentially expressed in healthy vs diabetic based on their fpkm value, graphical representation shows the variation in up and down regulation stream, more number of genes are observed in down regulation and comparatively very less number in up regulation are observed, which concludes the gene variation more in downstream process which has to be present at up regulationstream.

Table 20. Showing the numbers of genes differentially expressed in healthy and diabetic and variationsin up and down regulation

Genes	healthy vs prediabetic	healthy vs diabetic
DGE	3544	2306
UP	1597	497
DOWN	1948	1810

*DGE= Differential Gene Expression, UP=Upregulation, DR=Downregulation

Graph 7. Bar Graph showing the numbers of Genes differentially expressed in healthy , prediabetic anddiabetic, variations in UP and Down Regulation

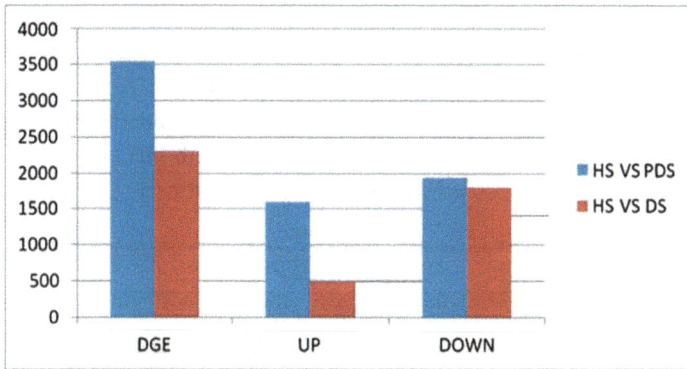

*HS=Healthy, PDS=Prediabetic, DS=Diabetic, DGE=Differential Gene Expression

Showing the comparative number of genes differentially expressed in healthy, prediabetic and diabetic focusing on up and down regulation, comparatively in healthy, prediabetic and diabetic indicates the up stream process with very less number of genes involvement using fpkm values, whereas most of the genes present in prediabetic and diabetic are found near about same in down stream, these fluctuations of genes in prediabetic and diabetic in up and down regulation indicates the metabolic and genetic variations in the studied subject.

Figure 13. *Hormonal (ligand) binding site and transcription process in nucleus*

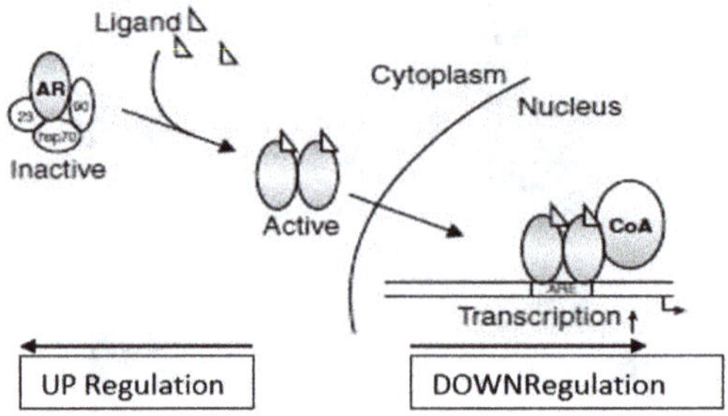

Showing the importance of activator, Receptor and repressor; a model applied to understand the receptors based on current molecular data, normally a inactive receptor is surrounded by specificproteins in the cytoplasm will be activated by the hormonal ligand and will be trasnlocated to thenucleus, binding to the DNA but also achieve the required bonding to nuclear proteins called activator, thus facilitating trancription (296). In type II diabetes, insulin is present and frequently levels are high, but patients have developed a resistance to insulin. The various explainations for this resistance include dysfunctional receptors, fatty aciDiabetic that interfere with binding or the absence of adiponectin (297).our study focused on Insulin Receptor Substrate (IRS).

Table 21. FPKM Value of top 25 genes in Upregulated Healthy, PreDiabetic and Diabetic Subject

FPKM_HEALTHY UR	FPKM_PREDIABETIC UR	FPKM DIABETIC UR
0.000317	0.100241	0.058094
0.000914	0.140528	1.207839
0.007074	1.044812	0.158297
0.002554	0.353901	0.519596
0.00532	0.721676	0.147916
0.015894	2.054316	0.145001
0.003747	0.475045	1.219037
0.01004	1.137538	0.1776
0.040882	4.150945	0.206711
0.010531	0.985301	0.284458
0.004543	0.411423	3.587456
0.008109	0.674661	0.260723
0.008401	0.659517	0.275949

0.013784	1.058291	0.314267
0.008213	0.600631	0.490089
0.021914	1.471149	0.957677
0.01652	1.04676	0.099589
0.050902	2.554587	0.436846
0.000336	0.015977	0.645853
0.006345	0.298815	0.315621
0.009833	0.448825	0.226789
0.007009	0.311309	0.460582
0.012146	0.515502	0.227246
0.049776	1.920783	3.085593
0.007683	0.290764	0.1776

Showing the FPKM value of selected top 25 genes values Log2FC > 0 of Upregulated genes in healthy,prediabetic and diabetic subjects.

Table 22. Comparison of Mean TOP 25 for Upregulated between two groups [Mann-Whitney U test]

	Mean±SD	Mann-Whitney U Value	P-value
FPKM_HEALTHY UR VS FPKM_PREDIABETIC UR	0.01661380±0.022317067 0.93402956±0.927404338	21.0	P<0.0001 S
FPKM_HEALTHY UR FPKM DIABETIC UR	0.01661380±0.022317067 0.62745716±0.876880380	10.00	P<0.0001S
FPKM_PREDIABETIC UR FPKM DIABETIC UR	0.93402956±0.927404338	201	P=0.031S

* HEALTHY= Healthy Subject, prediabetic= Prediabetic Subject, diabetic=Diabetic Subject, UR=UP regulated

Showing mann whitney u test for mean, standard deviation and p-vlaue, which signifies the normal distribution of the data in diabetic, prediabetic and healthy, where healthy subject mean is found to be optimum which indicates the availability of the receptor to act on and active the structureal genes on downregulation, whereas in pd subject it was observe more indication various receptors activated due to mutational, or snps process which was not required at that binding site, in diabetic subject also mutation has been observed which may effect the downregulation process.

p- value shows significance in healthy vs prediabetic, and in healthy vs diabetic, whereas some values has been increased while comparing prediabetic and diabetic and shows some significance too. mann whitney u test shows the unequal distribution in studied samples indicating alternative hypothesis.

Graph 8. Showing mean of top 25 upregulated genes in diabetic, prediabetic and healthy

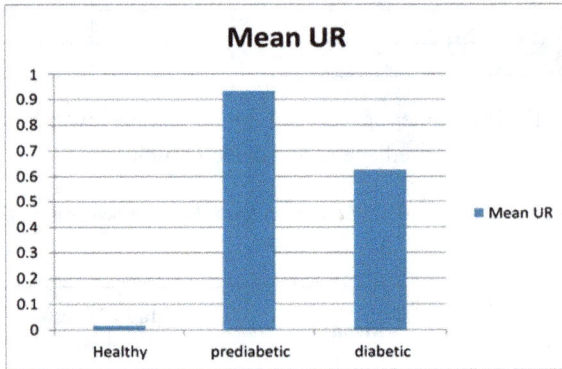

Graph showing the mean distribution of top 25 upregulated genes in diabetic, prediabetic and healthy samples where one can observe unequal distribution indicating the mutational changes in samples, whichdisturb the receptor mechanism and alter the transcription process in nucleus.

Table 23. Showing top 25 Downregulated Genes based on FPKM Value

FPKM_HEALTHY	FPKM_PREDIABETIC	FPKM_DIABETIC
0.766111	0.001295	0.000606
0.214053	0.001106	0.003582
0.199810	0.001218	0.000937
0.703186	0.004438	0.002119
0.933798	0.006299	0.003967
0.854285	0.006260	0.000509
0.350088	0.002590	0.004389
0.255243	0.002521	0.011002

106

0.745142	0.007438	0.005919
0.666154	0.006876	0.022165
0.450056	0.004979	0.007856
0.625753	0.007824	0.005042
0.163882	0.002300	0.006537
0.503446	0.007531	0.017757
0.826235	0.012710	0.006553
0.320117	0.005384	0.008637
0.920173	0.015510	0.002231
0.723536	0.012220	0.003220
0.368443	0.006305	0.007297
0.306915	0.005404	0.002646
0.477721	0.008765	0.024746
0.895945	0.017371	0.007388
1.580342	0.035571	0.005515
0.193351	0.004491	0.003867
0.449018	0.011278	0.014800

Showing the FPKM Values of the top 25 Genes Downregulated values log $2FC \leq 0$ in healthy, prediabetic and diabetic subjects

Table 24. Comparison of Mean TOP 25 for Downregulated between two groups [Mann-Whitney U test]

	Mean±SD	Mann-Whitney U Value	**P-value**
FPKM_HEALTHY DR VS FPKM_PREDIABETIC DR	0.56180320±0.347047164	**32.0**	**P<0.0001S**
	0.02581628±0.088449777		
FPKM_HEALTHY DR Vs FPKM DIABETIC DR	0.56180320±0.347047164	**9.00**	**P<0.0001S**
	0.00717148±0.006406731		
FPKM_PREDIABETIC DR Vs FPKM DIABETIC DR	0.02581628±0.088449777	**258**	**P=0.201NS**
	0.00717148±0.006406731		

* DR= DOWN regulated

Table showing the Mann Whitney U test for mean, Standard deviation, and P-vlaue of top 25 Downregullated genes, which signifies the normal distribution of the data in diabetic, prediabetic and healthy samples, in downregualtion healthy shows the mean value more as cpmared to prediabetic and diabetic, indicating the mutational effects on activating or enhancing the mrna in protein foramtion for the maintainence of the cell. p-value in downregulation shows the significance in healthy vs prediabetic and healthy vs prediabetic, whereas no significant shown in prediabetic vs diabetic population, showing uneual distribution indicating alternative hypothesis.

Graph 9. Showing mean of top 25 downregulated genes in diabetic, prediabetic and diabetic

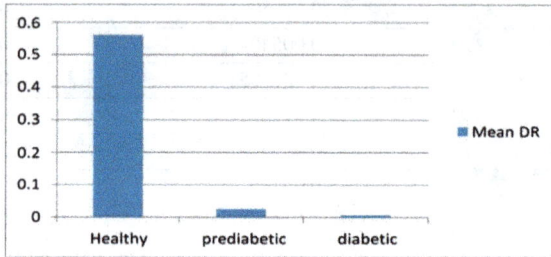

*DR=Downregulated

Graph showing the mean distribution of top 25 downregulated genes in diabetic, prediabetic and healthy samples where one can observe unequal distribution indicating the mutational changes in samples, whichdisturb the receptor mechanism and alter the transcription process in nucleus.

Graph 10. Comparative analysis of upregulated and downregulated genes (differential expressed genes) inhealthy, prediabetic and diabetic.

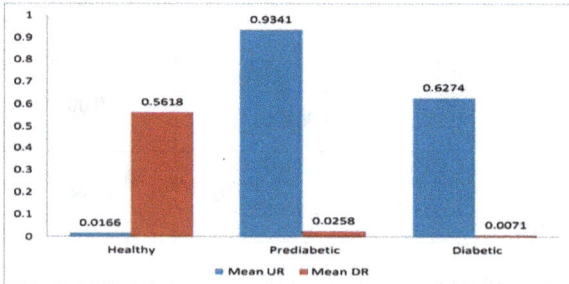

Graph indicating the comparative analysis of top 50 genes (25 up and 25 down) based on there fpkm values, mean values of top 50 genes indicates the drastic changes in transcription and translation process in studied samples which indicates the up and down regulation, at up regulation receptors has to be activated which led to produce and complete the process in down regulations to products which is required by the cell, here in prediabetic and diabetic huge amount of alteration due to SNPs, mutation or by pseudogene can be observed.

Table 25. Showing number of similar observed genes in healthy, prediabetic and diabetic

Title	Gene Numbers
genes which are expressed common in all subjects	4421
genes which are expressed common to healthy and prediabetic	2876
genes which are expressed common to healthy and diabetic	3163
genes which are expressed common to prediabeticand diabetic	470
number of genes expressed only in healthy	6444
number of genes expressed only in prediabetic	2193
number of genes expressed only in diabetic	2101

Graph 11. Number of genes expressed in studied subjects

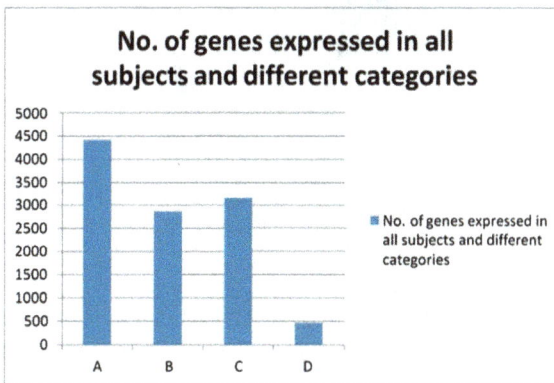

109

Showing the number of genes expressed in studied samples (healthy, prediabetic, and diabetic) bar diagram showing number of common genes expressed , a) showing the genes expressed in healthy, prediabetic and diabetic subject , b) shows the exclusively expressed gene in healthy and prediabetic, c) shows the exclusively expressed gene in healthy and diabetic, d) shows the exclusively expressed genein prediabetic and diabetic.

Graph 12. Number of genes expressed in Healthy, Prediabetic and Diabetic sample

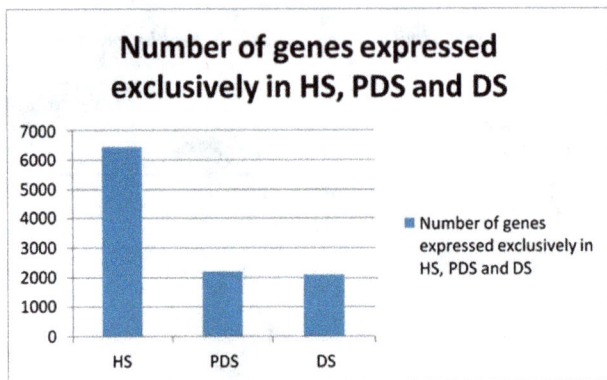

Figure 14. Venn diagram of all genes expressed in healthy, prediabetic and diabetic

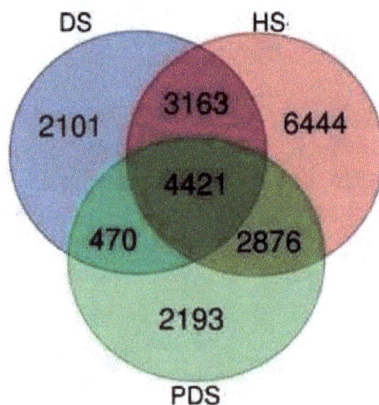

*HS= Healthy Subject, PDS= Prediabetic Subject, DS=Diabetic Subject

Venn Diagram representing a) common number of genes present in the healthy (pink color circle) 6444, prediabetic (green color circle) 2193, and diabetic (blue color circle)

110

2101, number of exclusively expressed genes in healthy (6444), prediabetic (2193) and diabetic (2101) samples, c) also number of common genes in healthy and prediabetic is 4421, and in healthy and diabetic is 3163 genes.

Gene Ontology(GO) analysis

The Gene Ontology project provides controlled vocabularies of defined terms representing gene product properties. These cover three domains: **Cellular Component**, the parts of a cell or its extracellular environment; **Molecular Function**, the elemental activities of a gene product at the molecular level, such as binding or catalysis; and **Biological Process**, operations or sets of molecular events with a defined beginning and end, pertinent to the functioning of integrated living units: cells, tissues, organs, and organisms. Gene Ontology analysis was performed by uploading the gene ID's on BioMart of all differentially expressed genes for all the 3 samples.

Figure 15. Gene ontology Biological Process in Healthy sample

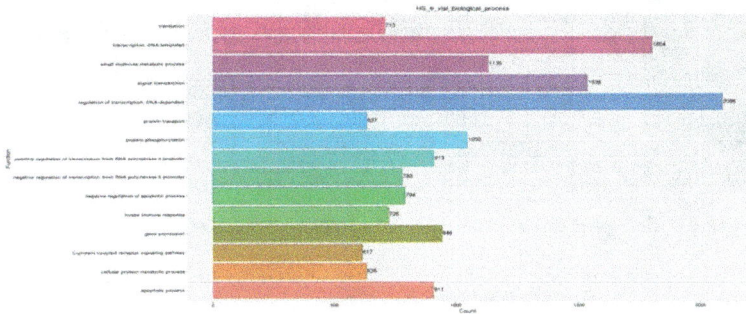

Figure 16. Gene Ontology Biological process in Prediabetic Sample

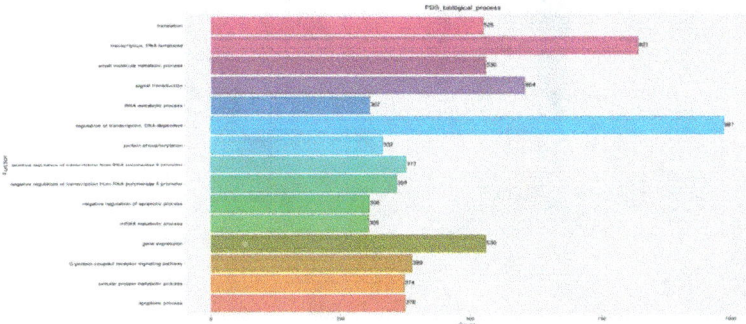

Figure 17. Gene ontology Biological Process in Diabetic sample

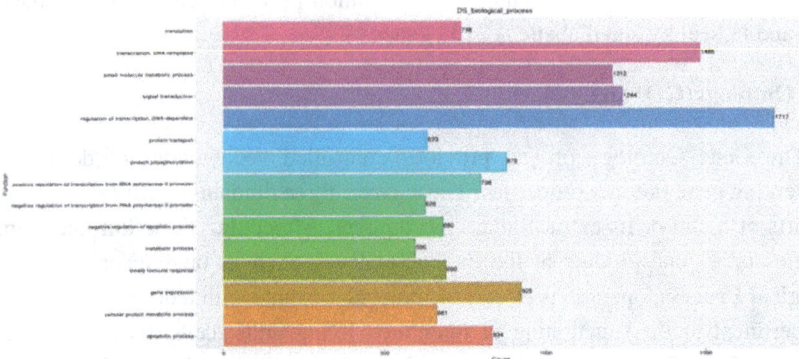

Table 26. Gene ontology Biological Process different function and their gene numbers in Healthy, Prediabetic and Diabetic sample

	translation	Signal Transduction	Protein Transport	Gene Expression	apoptotic process
Healthy	713	1538	637	946	911
Prediabetic	525	604	332	530	376
Diabetic	738	1244	633	925	834

Graph 13. Biological Process comparison in Healthy, prediabetic and diabetic sample

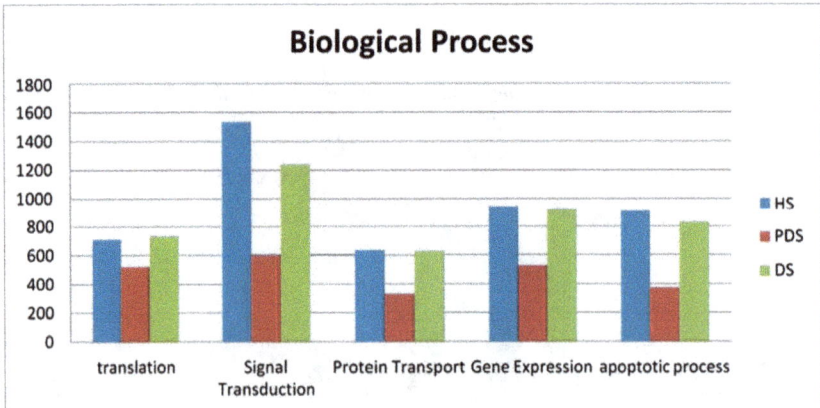

Showing the graphical representation of biological process in Gene ontology where different biological process (like: Translation, signal transduction, protein transport, gene expression, apoptotic process) are observed and the number of genes involved in it, which shows the variation/fluctuation in Prediabetic is less as compared to Healthy and Diabetic for cell regulation and maintenance.

Figure 18. Gene Ontology Cellular Processes in healthy Subject

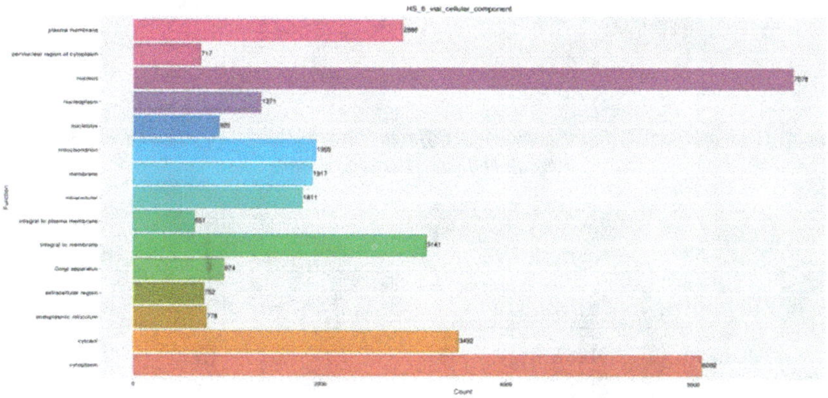

Figure 19. Gene Ontology Cellular Processes in Prediabetic Subject

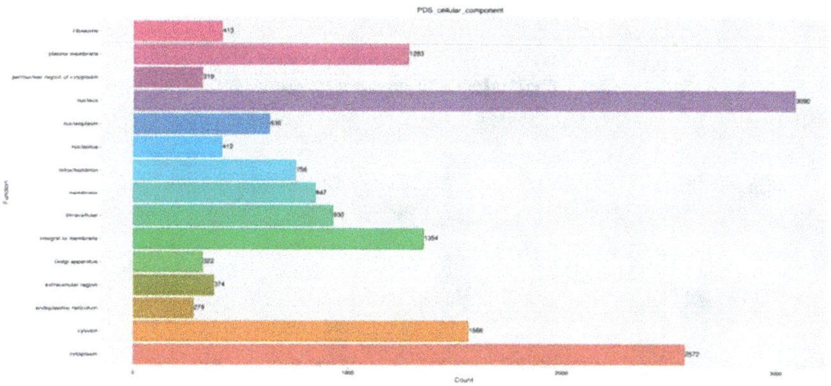

Figure 20. *Gene Ontology Cellular Processes in Diabetic Subject*

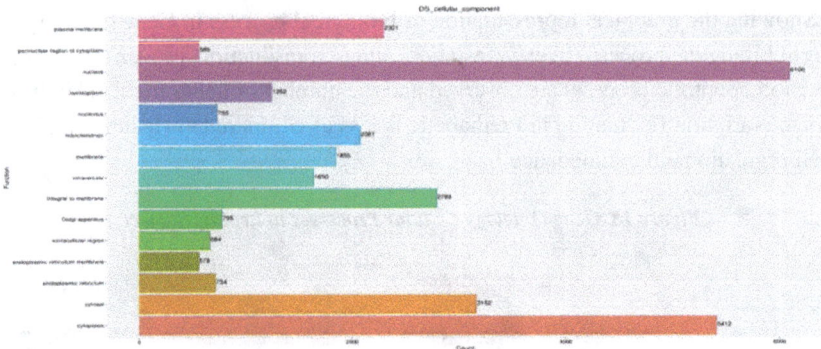

Table 27. Gene ontology Cellular component different function and their gene numbers inHealthy, Prediabetic and Diabetic sample

	Plasma membrane	Cytoplasm	Nucleus	Mitochondria	Golgi Apparatus
healthy	2886	717	7078	1955	974
prediabetic	1283	319	3090	756	322
diabetic	2301	585	6100	2081	795

Graph 14. Cellular Component in Healthy, Prediabetic and Diabetic sample

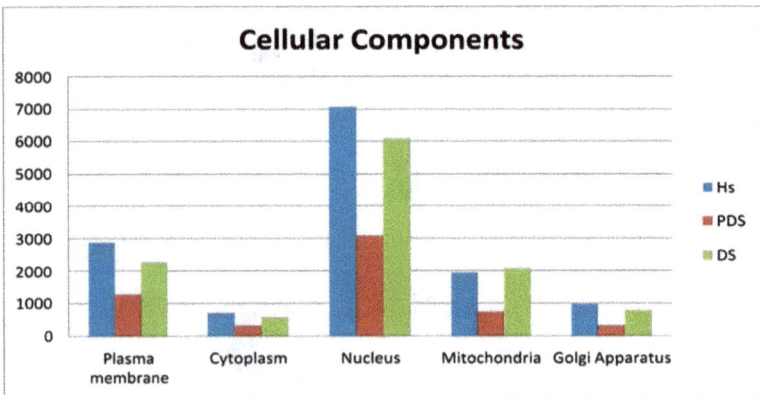

*HS= Healthy subject, PDS=Prediabetic subject, DS=Diabetic Subject

Showing the representation of gene ontology cellular components in healthy, prediabetic and diabetic sample where different cell components (like : Plasma membrane, cytoplasm, nucleus, mitochondria, Golgi apparatus and others) were observed the number of genes involved in it, where it shows thevarious fluctuation/ differences varied from healthy, to prediabetic and diabetic in golgi apparatusnumber of genes in prediabetic is very less (322) comparatively to diabetic (795) and Healthy (974) performing in Gene ontology.

Figure 21. Gene ontology molecular function in healthy sample

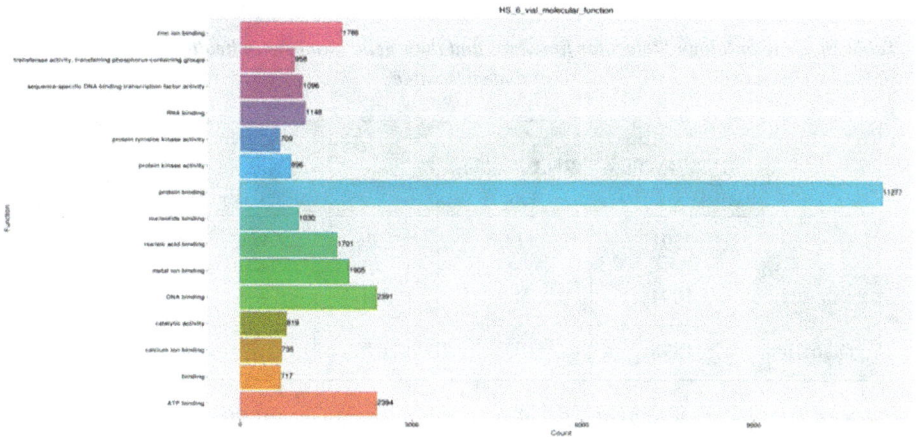

Figure 22. Gene ontology molecular function in prediabetic sample

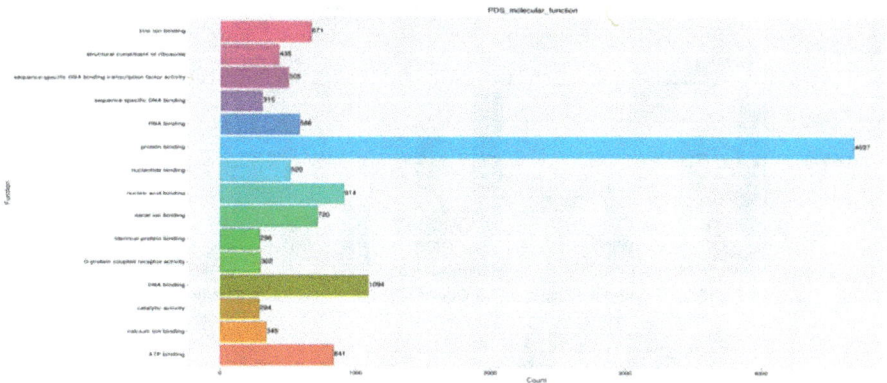

Figure 23. Gene ontology molecular function in diabetic sample

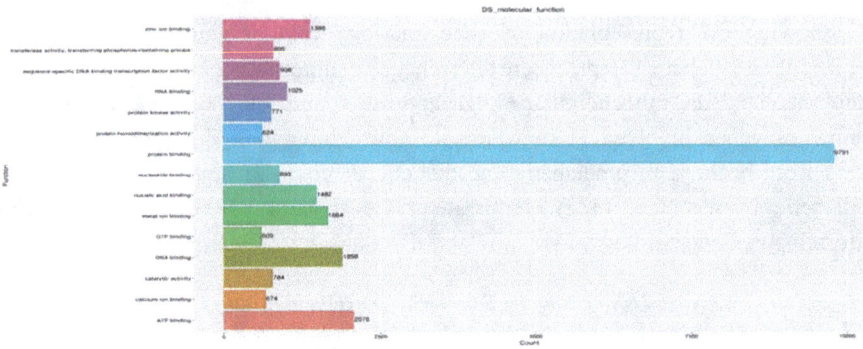

Table 28. Gene ontology Molecular functions and their gene numbers in healthy, prediabetic and diabeticsample

	DNA Binding	RNA Binding	ATP Binding	Protein Kinase activity	Catalytic Activity
Healthy	2391	1148	2394	896	819
Prediabetic	1094	586	841	296	294
Diabetic	1898	1025	2076	771	784

Graph 15. Gene ontology molecular functions and their gene numbers in Healthy, prediabetic and diabetic sample

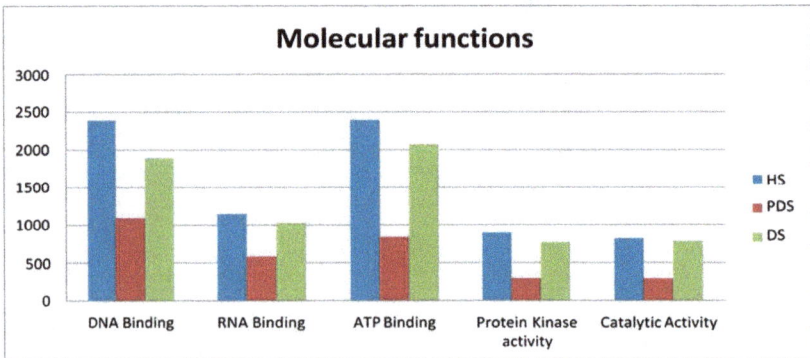

Shows the representation of genes number involved molecular function (like: DNA binding, RNAbinding, ATP binding, catalytic activity and others) in Gene ontology in Healthy, prediabetic and diabetic samples, which indicates the variants number of genes involved in healthy to prediabetic and diabetic, as observed in many molecular functions the involvement of genes found very less in prediabetic as compared to diabetic and healthy.

Pathway analysis

Ortholog assignment and mapping of the transcripts to the biological pathways were performed using **KEGG** automatic annotation server (**KAAS**). All the differentially expressed genes were compared against the KEGG database using BLASTX with threshold bit-score value of 60 (default). The mapped transcripts represented metabolic pathways of major Biomolecules such as carbohydrates, lipids, nucleotides, amino acids, glycans, cofactors, vitamins, terpenoids, polyketides, etc. The mapped genes also represented the genes involved in metabolism, genetic information processing, and environmental information processing and cellular processes.

Table 29. Distribution of gens in pathway analysis and categories across healthy, prediabetic and diabetic sample.

	healthy	prediabetic	diabetic	Total
Metabolism				
Carbohydrate metabolism	207	138	177	
Energy metabolism	187	142	185	
Lipid metabolism	181	102	153	
Nucleotide metabolism	132	92	101	
Amino acid metabolism	156	93	119	
Metabolism of other amino aciDiabetic	64	42	57	
Glycan biosynthesis and metabolism	124	76	97	
Metabolism of cofactors and vitamins	100	70	80	

Metabolism of terpenoiDiabetic and polyketides	17	13	19	
Biosynthesis of other secondarymetabolites	15	9	17	
Xenobiotics biodegradation andmetabolism	65	49	56	
Total	1248	826	1061	3135
Genetic Information Processing				
Transcription	234	136	209	
Translation	608	419	557	
Folding, sorting and degradation	392	227	351	
Replication and repair	135	71	87	
Membrane transport	23	13	13	
Signal transduction	896	566	706	
Signaling molecules and interaction	270	175	209	
Total	2558	1607	2132	6297
Cellular Processes				
Transport and catabolism	544	328	477	
Cell growth and death	458	265	375	
Cellular community - eukaryotes	250	159	180	
Cellular community - prokaryotes	7	4	5	
Cell motility	111	72	81	
Total	1370	828	1118	3316
Organismal Systems				
Immune system	649	404	548	
Endocrine system	432	275	367	

Circulatory system	129	90	114	
Digestive system	149	87	115	
Excretory system	73	46	67	
Nervous system	283	169	224	
Sensory system	362	221	142	
Development	159	90	118	
Aging	101	61	79	
Environmental adaptation	238	180	227	
Total	2575	1623	2001	6199
Human Diseases				
Cancers	626	419	541	
Immune diseases	218	153	201	
Neurodegenerative diseases	274	198	255	
Substance dependence	168	115	151	
Cardiovascular diseases	149	104	137	
Endocrine and metabolic diseases	292	207	268	
Infectious diseases	823	519	715	
Drug resistance	129	76	105	
Total	2679	1791	2373	6843
Grand Total	10430	6675	8794	

Showing the number of genes involved in different categories in cell regulations like human diseases, genetic information processes, cellular processes, metabolism etc are observed in healthy, prediabeticand diabetic samples where studied samples are mapped reference genome GrCh37.p13, indicates the mapped transcripts to the biological pathways, which have been performed using KEGG Server using BLASTX (Basic Local Alignment Search tool X (translated nucleotide to protein)), mapped transcripts number represent metabolic pathways of major Biomolecules such as carbohydrates, lipids, nucleotides, amino acids, co factor etc, also genes number involvement in genetic information processes, cellular processes, environmental information, human diseases etc.

Graph 16. Showing the number of genes involved in pathway analysis and categories in healthy, prediabetic and diabetic sample

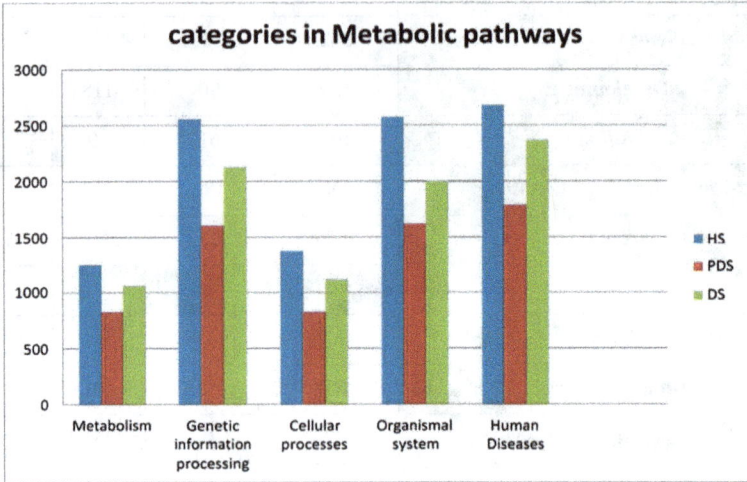

*HS= Healthy subject, PDS=Prediabetic subject, DS=Diabetic Subject

Showing the representation of gene number used different categories in Healthy, prediabetic and diabeticsample shown in table 28.

Table 30. Showing the numbe genes and its function working in glycolysis pathway in healthy subject

04930 Type II diabetes mellitus [PATH:ko04930]	Gene Card number	Functions
Healthy	K07187 IRS2	insulin receptor substrate 2
Healthy	K02649 PIK3R1_2_3	phosphoinositide-3-kinase regulatory subunitalpha/beta/delta
Healthy	K00922 PIK3CA_B_D	phosphatidylinositol-4,5-bisphosphate 3-kinase catalytic subunit alpha/beta/delta [EC:2.7.1.153]

120

Healthy	K00922 PIK3CA_B_D	phosphatidylinositol-4,5-bisphosphate 3-kinase catalytic subunit alpha/beta/delta [EC:2.7.1.153]
Healthy	K04371 MAPK1_3	mitogen-activated protein kinase 1/3 [EC:2.7.11.24]
Healthy	K07203 MTOR, FRAP, TOR	serine/threonine-protein kinase mTOR [EC:2.7.11.1]
Healthy	K04694 SOCS1, JAB	suppressor of cytokine signaling 1
Healthy	K04696 SOCS3, CIS3	suppressor of cytokine signaling 3
Healthy	K04697 SOCS4	suppressor of cytokine signaling 4
Healthy	K07209 IKBKB, IKKB	inhibitor of nuclear factor kappa-B kinase subunit beta [EC:2.7.11.10]
Healthy	K03156 TNF, TNFA	tumor necrosis factor superfamily, member 2
Healthy	K06068 PRKCD	novel protein kinase C delta type [EC:2.7.11.13]
Healthy	K07595 MAFA	transcription factor MAFA
Healthy	K00844 HK	hexokinase [EC:2.7.1.1]
Healthy	K00873 PK, pyk	pyruvate kinase [EC:2.7.1.40]
Healthy	K00873 PK, pyk	pyruvate kinase [EC:2.7.1.40]
Healthy	K05004 KCNJ11	potassium inwardly-rectifying channel subfamily J member 11
Healthy	K04851 CACNA1D	voltage-dependent calcium channel L type alpha-1D
Healthy	K04344 CACNA1A	voltage-dependent calcium channel P/Q typealpha-1A

Table showing the description of genes there name, number from gene card and their functions indicating the involvement of those genes in glycolysis in healthy sample.

Table 31. Showing the number genes and its function working in glycolysis pathway in Prediabetic Subject

04930 Type II diabetes mellitus [PATH:ko04930]	Gene Card number	Functions
Prediabetic	K17446 IRS4	insulin receptor substrate 4
Prediabetic	K00922 PIK3CA_B_D	phosphatidylinositol-4,5-bisphosphate 3-kinase catalytic subunit alpha/beta/delta [EC:2.7.1.153]
Prediabetic	K00922 PIK3CA_B_D	phosphatidylinositol-4,5-bisphosphate 3-kinase catalytic subunit alpha/beta/delta [EC:2.7.1.153]
Prediabetic	K00922 PIK3CA_B_D	phosphatidylinositol-4,5-bisphosphate 3-kinase catalytic subunit alpha/beta/delta [EC:2.7.1.153]
Prediabetic	K04696 SOCS3, CIS3	suppressor of cytokine signaling 3
Prediabetic	K07209 IKBKB, IKKB	inhibitor of nuclear factor kappa-B kinasesubunit beta [EC:2.7.11.10]
Prediabetic	K03156 TNF, TNFA	tumor necrosis factor superfamily, member 2
Prediabetic	K06068 PRKCD	novel protein kinase C delta type [EC:2.7.11.13]
Prediabetic	K18050 PRKCE	novel protein kinase C epsilon type[EC:2.7.11.13]
Prediabetic	K07595 MAFA	transcription factor MAFA
Prediabetic	K00844 HK	hexokinase [EC:2.7.1.1]
Prediabetic	K00873 PK, pyk	pyruvate kinase [EC:2.7.1.40]
Prediabetic	K00873 PK, pyk	pyruvate kinase [EC:2.7.1.40]
Prediabetic	K04851 CACNA1D	voltage-dependent calcium channel L typealpha-1D
Prediabetic	K04344 CACNA1A	voltage-dependent calcium channel P/Q type alpha-1A

Table showing the description of genes there name, number from gene card and their functionsindicating the involvement of those genes in glycolysis in Prediabetic sample.

Table 32. Showing the number genes and its function working in glycolysis pathway in diabetic Subject

04930 Type II diabetes mellitus [PATH:ko04930]	Gene card number	Functions
Diabetic	K07187 IRS2	insulin receptor substrate 2
Diabetic	K17446 IRS4	insulin receptor substrate 4
Diabetic	K02649 PIK3R1_2_3	phosphoinositide-3-kinase regulatory subunit alpha/beta/delta
Diabetic	K00922 PIK3CA_B_D	phosphatidylinositol-4,5-bisphosphate 3-kinase catalytic subunit alpha/beta/delta [EC:2.7.1.153]
Diabetic	K04371 MAPK1_3	mitogen-activated protein kinase 1/3 [EC:2.7.11.24]
Diabetic	K04694 SOCS1, JAB	suppressor of cytokine signaling 1
Diabetic	K04695 SOCS2, CIS2	suppressor of cytokine signaling 2
Diabetic	K04696 SOCS3, CIS3	suppressor of cytokine signaling 3
Diabetic	K07209 IKBKB, IKKB	inhibitor of nuclear factor kappa-B kinase subunit beta[EC:2.7.11.10]
Diabetic	K04440 JNK	c-Jun N-terminal kinase [EC:2.7.11.24]
Diabetic	K03156 TNF, TNFA	tumor necrosis factor superfamily, member 2
Diabetic	K06068 PRKCD	novel protein kinase C delta type [EC:2.7.11.13]
Diabetic	K07595 MAFA	transcription factor MAFA
Diabetic	K00844 HK	hexokinase [EC:2.7.1.1]
Diabetic	K00844 HK	hexokinase [EC:2.7.1.1]
Diabetic	K00844 HK	hexokinase [EC:2.7.1.1]
Diabetic	K00873 PK, pyk	pyruvate kinase [EC:2.7.1.40]
Diabetic	K05004 KCNJ11	potassium inwardly-rectifying channel subfamily J member 11
Diabetic	K04344 CACNA1A	voltage-dependent calcium channel P/Q type alpha-1A

Table showing the description of genes there name, number from gene card and their functions indicating the involvement of those genes in glycolysis in diabetic sample.

Figure 24. Graphical representation of enzyme used in Glycolysis pathway in Healthy Sample

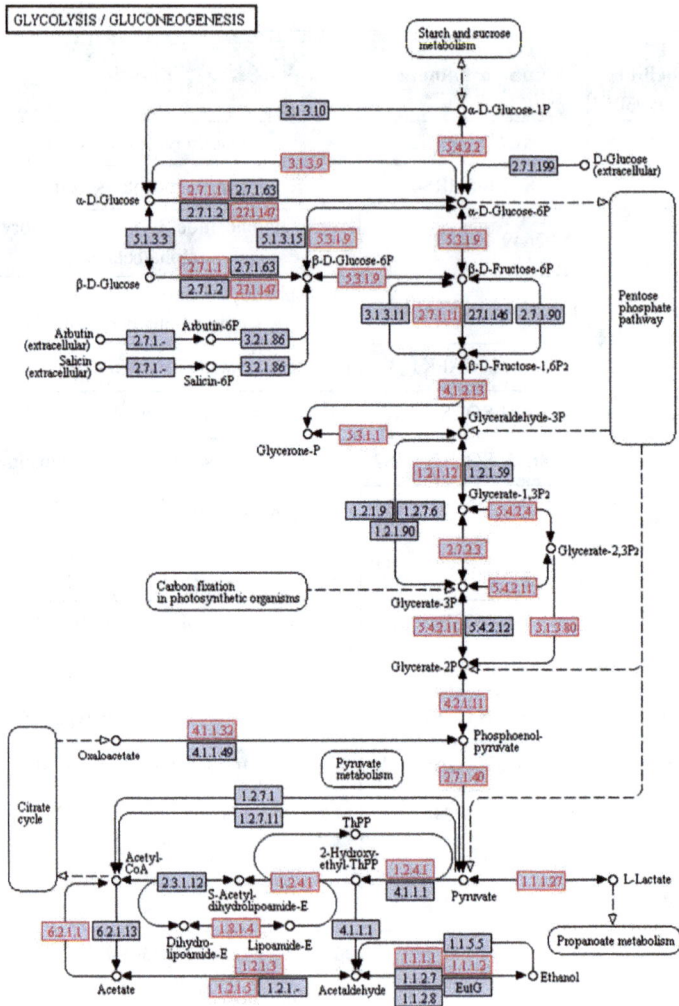

Figure 25. Graphical representation of enzyme used in Glycolysis pathway in Prediabetic Sample

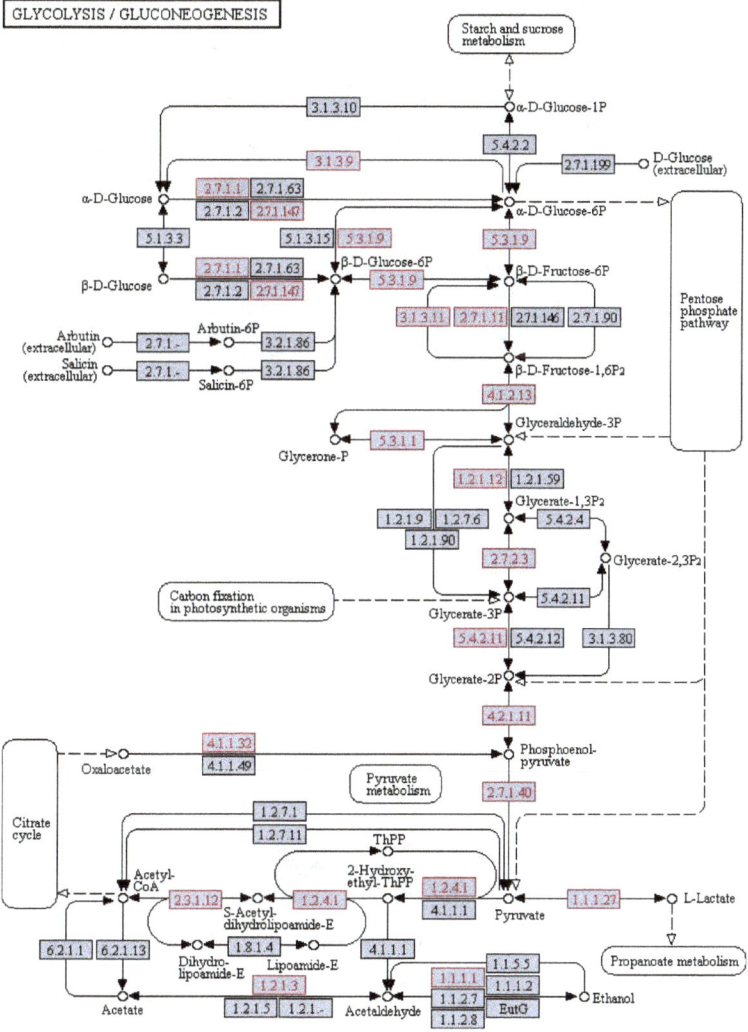

GLYCOLYSIS / GLUCONEOGENESIS

Starch and sucrose metabolism

3.1.3.10

α-D-Glucose-1P

5.4.2.2

3.1.3.9

2.7.1.199 → D-Glucose (extracellular)

α-D-Glucose

| 2.7.1.1 | 2.7.1.63 |
| 2.7.1.2 | 2.7.1.147 |

α-D-Glucose-6P

5.1.3.3   5.1.3.15   5.3.1.9   5.3.1.9

β-D-Glucose

| 2.7.1.1 | 2.7.1.63 |
| 2.7.1.2 | 2.7.1.147 |

β-D-Glucose-6P   5.3.1.9

β-D-Fructose-6P

Pentose phosphate pathway

Arbutin (extracellular)   2.7.1.-   Arbutin-6P   3.2.1.86

Salicin (extracellular)   2.7.1.-   Salicin-6P   3.2.1.86

3.1.3.11   2.7.1.11   2.7.1.146   2.7.1.90

β-D-Fructose-1,6P2

4.1.2.13

Glyceraldehyde-3P

5.3.1.1   Glycerone-P

1.2.1.12   1.2.1.59

Glycerate-1,3P2

1.2.1.9   1.2.7.6   5.4.2.4
1.2.1.90

2.7.2.3   Glycerate-2,3P2

Carbon fixation in photosynthetic organisms

5.4.2.11   Glycerate-3P

5.4.2.11   5.4.2.12   3.1.3.80

Glycerate-2P

4.2.1.11

4.1.1.32   Phosphoenol-pyruvate
4.1.1.49

Oxaloacetate

Pyruvate metabolism   2.7.1.40

Citrate cycle

1.2.7.1
1.2.7.11   ThPP

2-Hydroxy-ethyl-ThPP

Acetyl-CoA   2.3.1.12   S-Acetyl-dihydrolipoamide-E   1.2.4.1   1.2.4.1   1.1.1.27 → L-Lactate
4.1.1.1   Pyruvate

6.2.1.1   6.2.1.13   1.8.1.4   Dihydro-lipoamide-E   Lipoamide-E   4.1.1.1   Propanoate metabolism

1.2.1.3   1.1.5.5   1.1.1.1   1.1.1.2   EutG → Ethanol

Acetate   1.2.1.5   1.2.1.-   Acetaldehyde   1.1.2.7   1.1.2.8

125

Figure 26. Graphical representation of enzyme used in Glycolysis pathway in Diabetic Sample

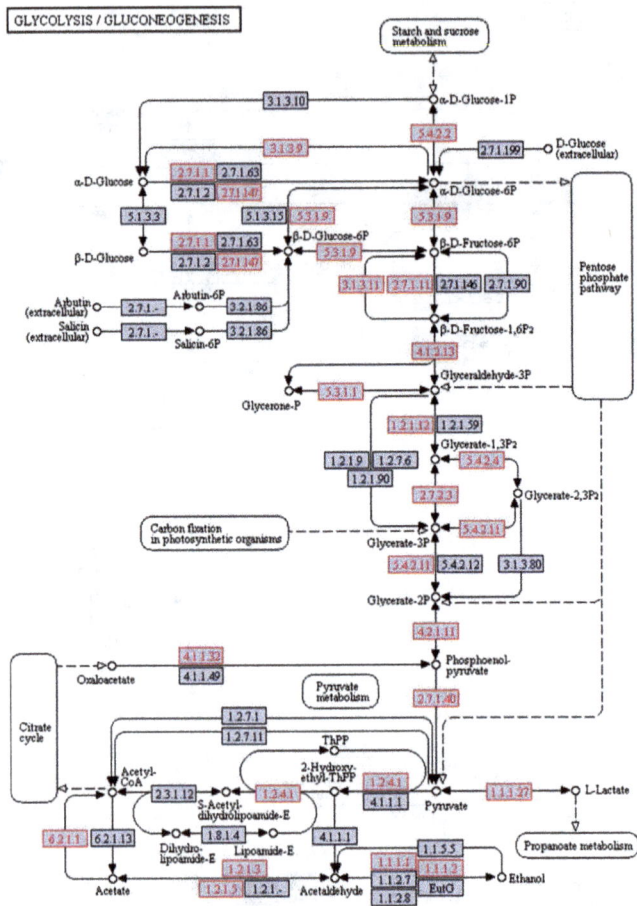

Figure 24, 25 and 26 represents the E.C (Enzyme Classification Number) of Enzymes which are expressed (blue boxed) in Healthy, prediabetic and diabetic sample which represents hyperlinked to ENZYME entries that are selected from the original version red box indicates the non expression hyperlinked to enzyme in glycolysis cycle.

⟶ Arrow indicates molecular interaction or relation between enzymes. ---► Arrow indicates indirect link or unknown reaction. Step by step process of enzyme interactions and indirect links are observed in healthy, prediabetic and diabetic sample.

Figure 27. Graphical representation of Citrate Cycle (TCA cycle) in Healthy Subject

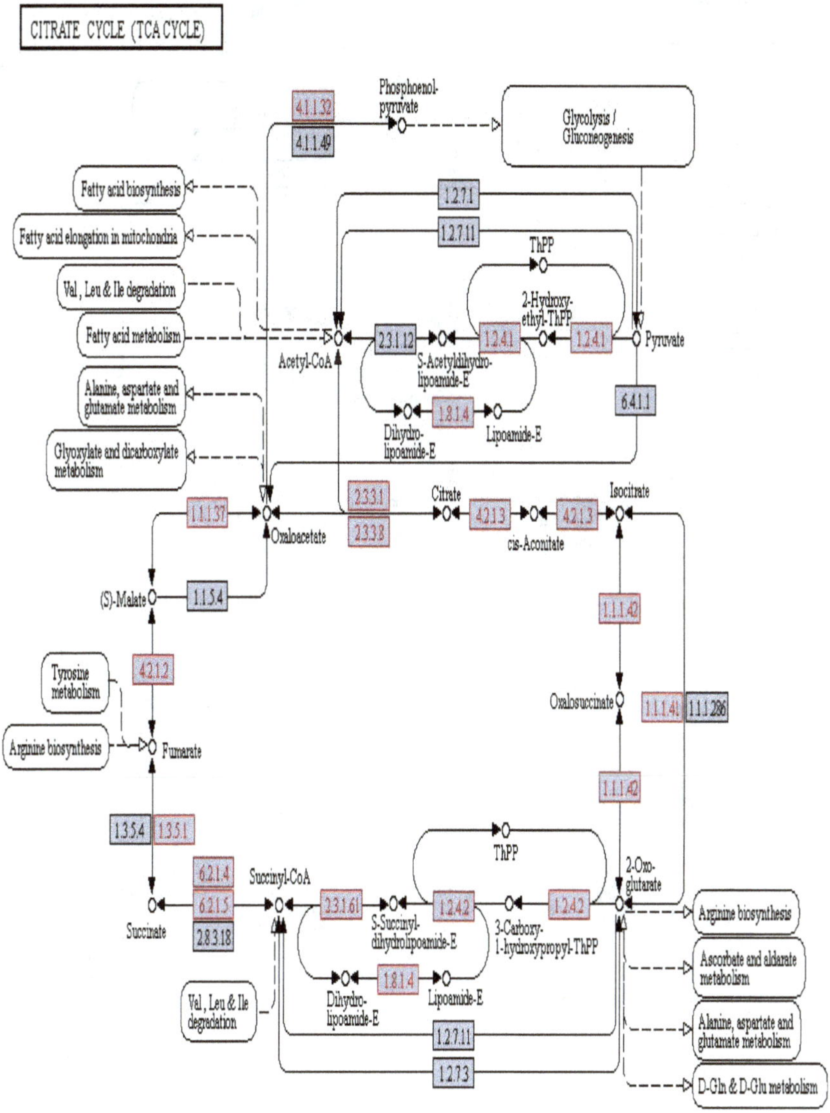

Figure 28. Graphical representation of Citrate Cycle (TCA cycle) in Prediabetic Subject

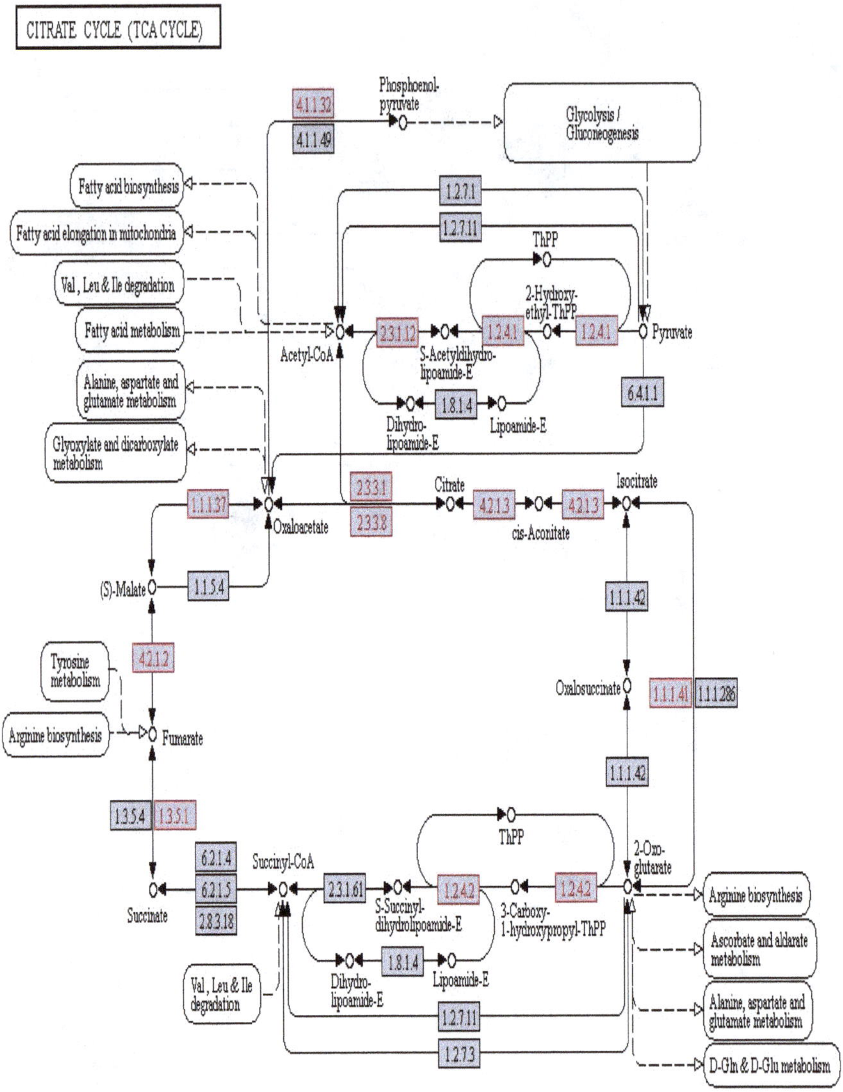

CITRATE CYCLE (TCA CYCLE)

128

Figure 29. Graphical representation of Citrate Cycle (TCA cycle) in Diabetic Subject

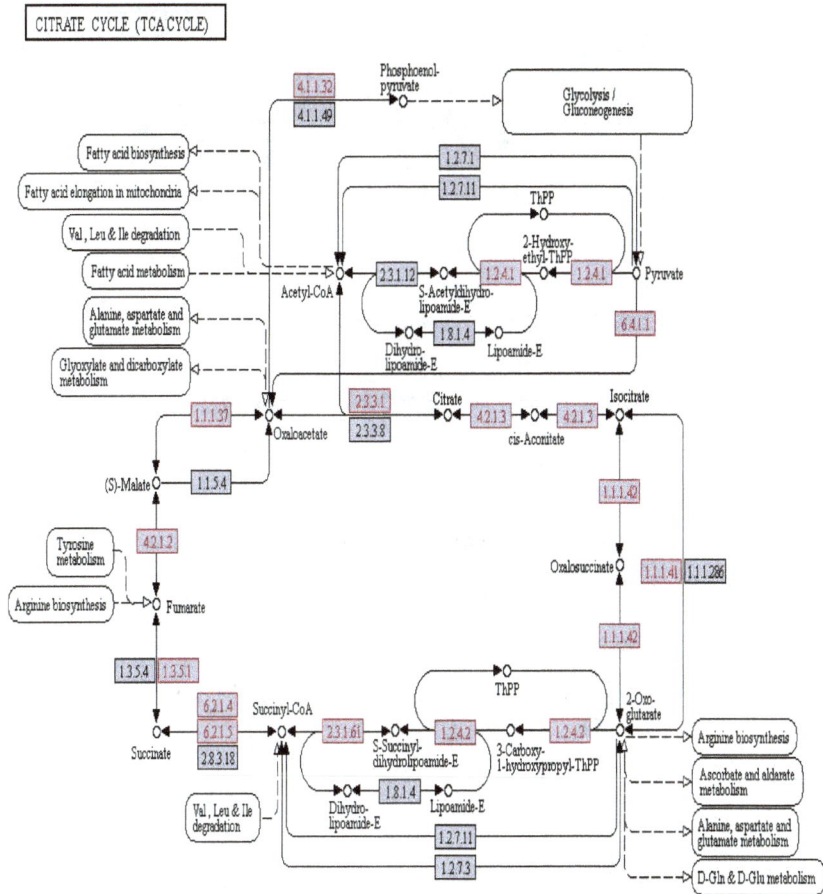

Figure no 27, 28 and 29 E.C number (Enzyme Classification) of Tricarboxylic Cycle (TCA cycle) are observed in Healthy, prediabetic and diabetic samples where blue box indicate hyperlinked to enzyme reaction that are selected to original version where red box indicates the non expression of the enzyme reaction in said metabolic pathway. ⟶ Arrow indicates molecular interaction or relation between enzymes. ---► Arrow indicates indirect link or unknown reaction. Step by step process of enzyme interactions and indirect links are observed in healthy, prediabetic and diabetic sample.

129

Figure 30. Oxidative Phosphorylation cycle in Healthy sample

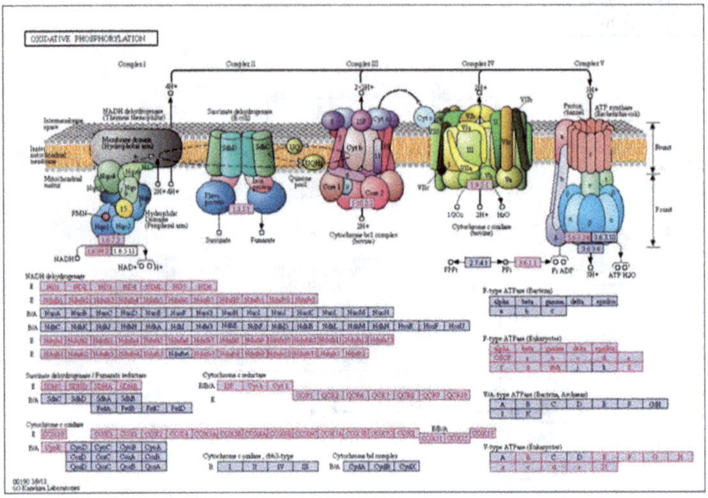

Figure 31. Oxidative phosphorylation cycle in Prediabetic sample

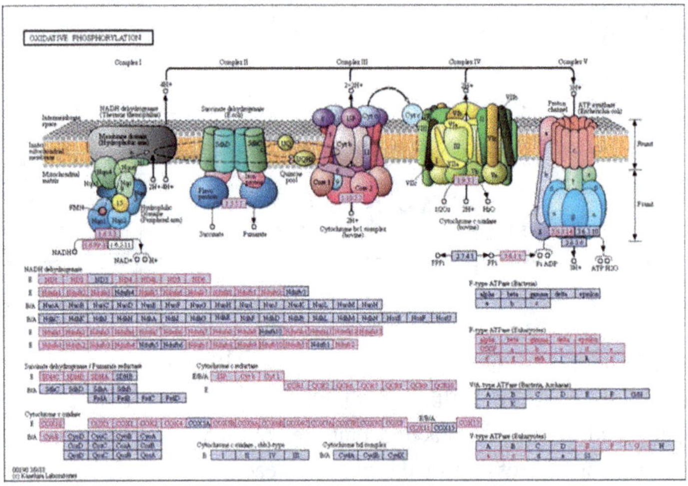

Figure 32. Oxidative Phosphorylation cycle in Diabetic Sample

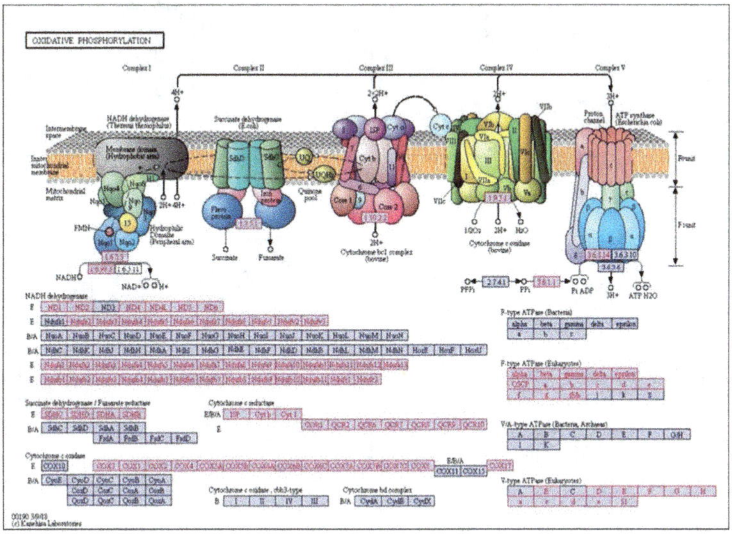

Figure 30, 31 and 32 shows the KEGG Pathway diagram of Healthy, prediabetic and diabetic samples including the oxidative phosphorylation system (OXPHOS) genes selected by transcriptome (Microarray analysis). In all 3 diagram upper part shows the respiratory chain complex with the corresponding Enzyme classification (E.C) number are observed. In bottom, rectangles indicating the subunits of each respiratory chain complex. The subunits encoded by genes analysed by transcriptome are shown in black colored rectangle.

Table 33. Showing the different classes of enzyme and genes involvement comparatively studied in glycolysis pathway in healthy, prediabetic and diabetic

Entry	Name	Class	Substrate	Product	Comment	Pathways	Genes
1.1.1.2	Alcohol dehydrogenase (NADP)	Oxidoreductase	Alcohol, NADP+	Aldehyde, NADPH	Off in PREDIA BETIC	Glycolysis, gluconeogenesis	HSA, PTS, PPr, GGO, PON, NLE, MCC, MCF, CASB, RRO
3.13.8.0	MIPP1	Hydrolases	2,3-bisphospho-D-Glycerate	2-phospho-D-glycerate	Off in PREDIA BETIC and DIABETIC	Glycolysis, gluconeogenesis	HSA, PTS, PPr, GGO, PON, NLE, MCC, MCF, CASB, RRO
5.4.2.11	Phosphoglycerate Mutase	Isomerases	2-phospho-D-Glycerate	3-phodpho-D-Glycerate	Off in PREDIA BETIC	Glycolysis, gluconeogenesis	HAS, PTS, PPr, GGO, PON, NLE, MCC, MCF, CASB, RRO
2.3.1.12	Dihydrolipoyll ysine-residue acetyltransferase	Transferase	AcetylCoA	CoA	Off in HEALTHY and DIABETIC	Glycolysis, gluconeogenesis	HAS, PTS, PPr, GGO, PON, NLE, MCC, MCF, CASB, RRO
1.2.1.5	Aldehyde Dehydrogenase	Oxidoreductase	Aldehyde, NAD+, NADP+	Carboxylate, NADH and NADPH	Off in PREDIA BETIC	Glycolysis, gluconeogenesis	HAS, PTS, PPr, GGO, PON, NLE, MCC, MCF, CASB, RRO

EC Number	Enzyme	Class	Substrate	Product	Status	Pathway	Organisms
5.4.2.2	Phosphogluco mutase	Isomerase	Aplha-D-Glucose-Phosphate	D-Glucose6-Phosphate	Off in PREDIA BETIC	Glycolysis, gluconeogenesis	HAS, PTS, PP, GGO, PON, NLE, MCC, MCF, CASB, RRO
3.1.3.11	Fructose Diphosphate	Hydrolase	D-Fructose-1,6-Bisphosphate	D-Fructose6 phosphate	Off in HEALTH Y	Glycolysis, gluconeogenesis	HAS, PTS, PP, GGO, PON, NLE, MCC, MCF, CASB, RRO
6.2.1.1	Acetate CoA ligase, synthetase	Ligases (forming C-S bond	ATP, Acetate, CoA	AMP, Acetyl-CoA	Off in PREDIA BETIC	Glycolysis, gluconeogenesis	HAS, PTS, PP, GGO, PON, NLE, MCC, MCF, CASB, RRO
1.8.1.4	Dihydrolipoyl dehydrogenase	Oxidoreductase	Protein N6-(dihydrolipoyl) lysine	ProteinN6-lipoyllysine, NADH	Off in PREDIA BETIC and DIABETIC	Glycolysis, gluconeogenesis	HAS, PTS, PP, GGO, PON, NLE, MCC, MCF, CASB, RRO

Listed Enzymes classification observed from Kyoto Encyclopedia of Genes and Genome (KEGG) utilised in GlycolysisCycle observed in Healthy, prediabetic and diabetic sample.

Graph 17. Number of genes obseved in healthy, prediabetic and diabetic

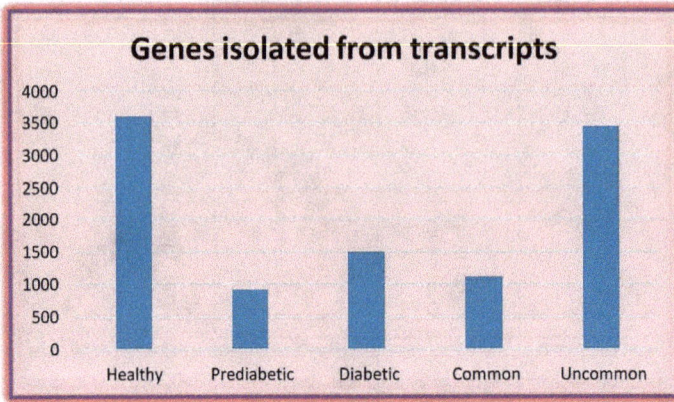

Graph 17. Number of genes obseved in healthy, prediabetic and diabetic

Showing the number of differential gene expressed in healthy, prediabetic and diabetic sample where also number of common and uncommon genes which are observed in studied sample, variant amount of gene numbers are observed which shows the variation in general respectively in the sample, and also vast difference in common and uncommon socket.

Some examples of fasta transcript sequence obtained after transcriptome sequencing, down and up regulated fragrments have been shortlisted from top 25 genes, from healthy, prediabetic and diabetic samples , where SNPs (Single nucleotide polymorphism) and Psuedogenes have been observed and those obtained fasta sequence has been processed and there structural parameters have been studied likeQ-MEAN (graph 17), which shows the structural modification based on genetic alteration in the sequence.

a) Located on chromosome 12 Downregulated (function:- protein jjunctional adhesion molecule, counter receptor for JAM2 gene, mediating leukocyte-platelet interaction as involved in the regulation of transepithelial migration of polymorphonuclear neutrophils, also play important role in angiogenesis).

>DIABETIC.14871.2 gene=DIABETIC.14871 reference_id=ENST00000593589 ref_gene_id=ENSG00000230291ref_gene_name=RP11-244J10.1cov=0.221219FPKM= 0.030998TPM=0.023477

Diabetic Subject DIABETIC

ATGAAGTTTAATCCCTTTGTGACTTCCGACCGAAGCAAGAATCGCAAAAGGC
ATTTCAACGCACCTTCCCACATTCGAAGGAAGATTATGTCTTCCCTTCTTTCC
AAAGAGCTGAGACAGAAGTACAACGAGCGATCCATGCCCATCCGAAAGGAC
GATGAAGTTCAGGTTGTACGAGGACACTACGAAGGTCAGCAAATTGGCAAA
GTGGTCCAGGTTTACAGGAAGAAATATGTTATCTACATTGAATGGGTGCAGC
GGGAAAAGGCTAATGGCACAACTGTCCACATAGGCATTCACTCCAGCAAGG
TGGTTATCACTAGGCTAAAACTGGACAAAGACAGCAAAAAGATCCTTGAAC
GGAAAGCCAAATCTCGCCAAGTAGGAAAGGAAAAGGGCAAATACAAGGAG
AAACAATTGAGAAGATGGAGGAATAA

Table 34. Showing the Open Reading Frame (ORF) ENSG00000230291 of healthy sample

5'3' Frame 1
Met K F N P F V T S D R S K N R K R H F N A P S H I R R K I Met S S L L S K E L R Q K Y N E
R S Met P I R K D D E V Q V V R G H Y E G Q Q I G K V V Q V Y R K K Y V I Y I E W V Q R E K
A N G T T V H I G I H S S K V V I T R L K L D K D S K K I L E R K A K S R Q V G K E K G K Y
K E E T I E K Met E E Stop

5'3' Frame 2
Stop S L I P L Stop L P T E A R I A K G I S T H L P T F E G R L C L P F F P K S Stop D R S T T S
D P C P S E R T Met K F R L Y E D T T K V S K L A K W S R F T G R N Met L S T L N G C S G K R
L Met A Q L S T Stop A F T P A R W L S L G Stop N W T K T A K R S L N G K P N L A
K Stop E R K R A N T R K K Q L R R W R N

5'3' Frame 3
E V Stop S L C D F R P K Q E S Q K A F Q R T F P H S K E D Y V F P S F Q R A E T E V Q R A I
H A H P K G R Stop S S G C T R T L R R S A N W Q S G P G L Q E E I C Y L H Stop Met G A A G K
G Stop W H N C P H R H S L Q Q G G Y H Stop A K T G Q R Q Q K D P Stop T E S Q I S P S R K
G K G Q I Q G R N N Stop E D G G I

3'5' Frame 1
L F L H L L N C F F L V F A L F L S Y L A R F G F P F K D L F A V F V Q F Stop P S D N H L A
G V N A Y V D S C A I S L F P L H P F N V D N I F L P V N L D H F A N L L T F V V S S Y N L N
F
I V L S D G H G S L V V L L S Q L F G K K G R H N L P S N V G R C V E Met P F A I L A S V G
S T K G M Q L H

3'5' Frame 2
Y S S I F S I V S S L Y L P F S F P T W R D L A F R S R I F L L S L S S F S L V I T T L L
E Stop Met P Met W T V V P L A F S R C T H S Met Stop I T Y F F L Stop T W T T L P I C Stop P
S Stop C P R T T Stop T S S S F R L Y F C L S S L E R R E D I I F L R Met W
E G A L K C L L R F L L R S E V T K G L N F

135

I P P S S Q L F L P C I C P F P F L L G E I W L S V Q G S F C C L C P V L A Stop Stop Stop P P C W S E C L C G Q L C H Stop P F P A A P I Q C R Stop H I S S C K P G P L C Q F A D L R S V L L H R P E G W A W I A R C T S V S A L Met G Met D R S P S S F E C G K V R Stop N A F C D S C F G R K S Q R D Stop T S

>PREDIABETIC.92290.1gene=PREDIABETIC.92290reference_id=ENST000004 92623ref_gene_id=ENSG00000230291 ref_gene_name=RP11-244J10.1 cov=4.634483 FPKM=0.870491TPM=0.581564

Prediabetic Subject PREDIABETIC

ATGAAGTTTAATCCCTTTGTGACTTCCGACCGAAGCAAGAATCGCAAAAGGC
ATTTCAACGCACCTTCCCACATTCGAAGGAAGATTATGTCTTCCCTTCTTTCC
AAAGAGCTGAGACAGAAGTACAACGAGCGATCCATGCCCATCCGAAAGGAC
GATGAAGTTCAGGTTGTACGAGGACACTACGAAGGTCAGCAAATTGGCAAA
GTGGTCCAGGTTTACAGGAAGAAATATGTTATCTACATTGAATGGTGCAGCG
GGAAAAGGCTAATGGCACAACTGTCCACATAGGCATTCACTCCAGCAAGGT
GGTTATCACTAGGCTAAAACTGGACAAAGACAGCAAAAAGATCCTTGAACG
GAAAGCCAAATCTCGCCAAGTAGGAAAGGAAAAGGGCAAATACAAGGAAG
AAACAATTGAGAAGATGGAGGAA

Table 35. Showing the Open Reading Frame (ORF) ENSG00000230291 of Prediabetic sample

5'3' Frame 1

Met K F N P F V T S D R S K N R K R H F N A P S H I R R K I Met S S L L S K E L R Q K Y N E R S Met P I R K D D E V Q V V R G H Y E G Q Q I G K V V Q V Y R K K Y V I Y I E W V Q R E K A N G T T V H I G I H S S K V V I T R L K L D K D S K K I L E R K A K S R Q V G K E K G K Y K E E T I E K Met E E

5'3' Frame 2

Stop S L I P L Stop L P T E A R I A K G I S T H L P T F E G R L C L P F F P K S Stop D R S T T S D P C P S E R T Met K F R L Y E D T T K V S K L A K W S R F T G R N Met L S T L N G C S G K R L Met A Q L S T Stop A F T P A R W L S L G Stop N W T K T A K R S L N G K P N L A K Stop E R K R A N T R K K Q L R R W R

5'3' Frame 3

E V Stop S L C D F R P K Q E S Q K A F Q R T F P H S K E D Y V F P S F Q R A E T E V Q R A I H A H P K G R Stop S S G C T R T L R R S A N W Q S G P G L Q E E I C Y L H Stop Met G A A G K G Stop W H N C P H R H S L Q Q G G Y H Stop A K T G Q R Q Q K D P Stop T E S Q I S P S R K G K G Q I Q G R N N Stop E D G G

136

3'5' Frame 1
F L H L L N C F F L V F A L F L S Y L A R F G F P F K D L F A V F V Q F **Stop** P S D N H L A G VN A Y V D S C A I S L F P L H P F N V D N I F L P V N L D H F A N L L T F V V S S Y N L N F I V L S D G H G S L V V L L S Q L F G K K G R H N L P S N V G R C V E **Met** P F A I L A S V G S H K G I K L H

3'5' Frame 2
S S I F S I V S S L Y L P F S F P T W R L **Met** G **Met** D R S . L S L S S F S L V I T T L L E **Stop** **Met** P **Met** W T V V P L A F S R C T H S **Met** Stop I T Y F F L **Stop** T W T T L P I C **Stop** P S **Stop** C P R T T **Stop** T S S S F R L Y F C L S S L E R R E D I I F L R **Met** W E G A L K C L L R F L L R S E V T K G L N F

3'5' Frame 3
P P S S Q L F L P C I C P F P F L L G E I W L S V Q G S F C C L C P V L A **Stop Stop Stop** P P C WS E C L C G Q L C H **Stop** P F P A A P I Q C R **Stop** H I S S C K P G P L C Q F A D L R S V L V Q PEL H R P F G W A W I A R C T S V S A L W K E G K T **Stop** S S F E C G K V R **Stop** N A F C D S C F G R K S Q R D **Stop** T S

>HEALTHY-6_vial.108899.2gene=healthy-6_vial.108899reference_id=ENST000
00593589ref_gene_id=ENSG00000230291ref_gene_name=RP11-244J10.1cov=0.2161
16FPKM=0.037963TPM=0.036607

Healthy Subject HEALTHY

ATGAAGTTTAATCCCTTTGTGACTTCCGACCGAAGCAAGAATCGCAAAAGGC
ATTTCAACGCACCTTCCCACATTCGAAGGAAGATTATGTCTTCCCTTCTTTCC
AAAGAGCTGAGACAGAAGTACAACGAGCGATCCATGCCCATCCGAAAGGAC
GATGAAGTTCAGGTTGTACGAGGACACTACGAAGGTCAGCAAATTGGCAAA
GTGGTCCAGGTTTACAGGAAGAAATATGTTATCTACATTGAATGGGTGCAGC
GGGAAAAGGCTAATGGCACAACTGTCCACATAGGCATTCACTCCAGCAAGG
TGGTTATCACTAGGCTAAAACTGGACAAAGACAGCAAAAAGATCCTTGAAC
GGAAAGCCAAATCTCGCCAAGTAGGAAAGGAAAAGGGCAAATACAAGGAA
GAAACAATTGAGAA GATGGAGGAATAA

Table 36. Showing the Open Reading Frame (ORF) ENSG00000230291 of diabetic sample

5'3' Frame 1
Met K F N P F V T S D R S K N R K R H F N A P S H I R R K I Met S S L L S K E L R Q K Y N E R S Met P I R K D D E V Q V V R G H Y E G Q Q I G K V V Q V Y R K K Y V I Y I E W V Q R E K A N G T T V H I G I H S S K V V I T R L K L D K D S K K I L E R K A K S R Q V G K E K G K Y K E E T I E K Met E E Stop

5'3' Frame 2
Stop S L I P L Stop L P T E A R I A K G I S T H L P T F E G R L C L P F F P K S Stop D R S T T S D P C P S E R T Met K F R L Y E D T T K V S K L A K W S R F T G R N Met L S T L N G C S G K R L Met A Q L S T Stop A F T P A R W L S L G Stop N W T K T A K R S L N G K P N L A K Stop E R K R A N T R K K Q L R R W R N

5'3' Frame 3
E V Stop S L C D F R P K Q E S Q K A F Q R T F P H S K E D Y V F P S F Q R A E T E V Q R A I H A H P K G R Stop S S G C T R T L R R S A N W Q S G P G L Q E E I C Y L H Stop Met G A A G K G Stop W H N C P H R H S L Q Q G G Y H Stop A K T G Q R Q Q K D P Stop T E S Q I S P S R K G K G Q I Q G R N N Stop E D G G I

3'5' Frame 1
L F L H L L N C F F L V F A L F L S Y L A R F G F P F K D L F A V F V Q F Stop P S D N H L A G V N A Y V D S C A I S L F P L H P F N V D N I F L P V N L D H F A N L L T F V V S S Y N L N F I V L S D G H G S L V V L L S Q L F G K K G R H N L P S N V G R C V E Met P F A I L A S V G S H K G I K L H

3'5' Frame 2
Y S S I F S I V S S L Y L P F S F P T W R D L A F R S R I F L L S L S S F S L V I T T L L E Stop Met P Met W T V V P L A Stop I T Y F F L Stop T W T T L P I C Stop P S Stop C P R T T Stop T S S S F R L Y F C L S S L E R R E D I I F L R Met W E G A L K C L L R F L L R S E V T K G L N F

3'5' Frame 3
I P P S S Q L F L P C I C P F P F L L G E I W L S V Q G S F C C L C P V L A Stop Stop Stop P P C W S E C L C G Q L C H Stop P F P A A P I Q C R Stop H I S S C K P G P L C Q F A D L R S V L V Q P E L H R P F G W A W I A R C T S V S A L W K E G K T Stop S S F E C G K V R Stop N A F C D S C F G R K S Q R D Stop T S

Table 37. Single nucleotide Polymorphism (SNPs)

Subject	SNP
Healthy	GG**AAT**AA
Prediabetic	GG**AGG**AA
Diabetic	GG**AAT**AA

Single nucleotide polymorphism fragment observed in healthy, prediabetic and diabetic fragment, showing Six frame translation the nucleotide sequence is shown in the middle with forward transaltion above and reverse translation below, two to three possible open reading frames with the sequence are highlighted.

Table 38. E-value and Q-Mean (Qualitative Model Energy Analysis) protein structure of fragmentin Healthy, prediabetic and diabetic sample

Sr. No.	Description	E-Value	QMEAN	Protein Structure	Uniprot Accession
1.	Healthy Sequence from chromosome 12P	8.2E-30	-1.02		A0A024RBF6 (A0A024RBF6_HUMAN)
2.	Pre-Diabetic from chromosome 12P	2.5E-29	-2.79		A0A024RBF6 (A0A024RBF6_HUMAN)

3.	Diabetic Sequence from chromosome 12P	1.9E-30	-2.78		A0A024RBF6 (A0A024RBF6_HUMAN)

Table showing E-Value (Similarity) Q mean (degree of nativeness) result and protein structure molecule, α helix, β sheat, and turn description and observed variants found in Prediabetic and diabetic compared with Healthy also structural loop (Blue color turn) can be seen in healthy where as one loop is missing in prediabetic and diabetic fragment absence of Glutamine (charged neutral polar amino acid), and aspargine (polar aliphatic amino acid) also dark blue colour loop in left hand side of the picture is missing in Prediabetic and diabetic samples structure, which indicates the absence of tyrosine (occurs in proteins that are part of signal transduction processes and functions as a receiver of phosphate groupsthat are transferred by way of protein kinases) and phenylalanine (Phenylalanine is a precursorfor tyrosine) in the structure.

Graph 18. Q- Mean value in Healthy, prediabetic and Diabetic

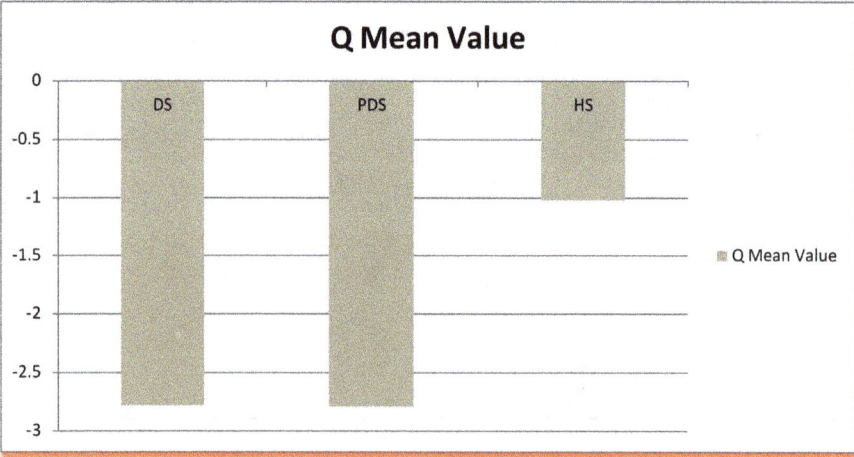

*DS=Diabetic, PDS=Prediabetic, HS=Healthy Subjects

Graph showing QMEAN and agreement terms range from 0 to 1 and the statistical potential termsdeliver pseudo energies with **negative values for energetically favourable states**. In the Z-score calculations, we adjusted the sign of the statistical terms such that higher Z-score consistently relate to favourable states, i.e. **higher QMEAN Z-score means better agreement** with predicted features and **lower mean force potential energy**. Value nearer to – (minus) one is observed in healthy whereas diabetic and prediabetic tends to be – (minus) 2.79, and 2.78 respectively.

b) Located on Chromosome 6 upregulated (processed pseudogene:- The processed pseudogenes reportedto date fall into three categories: those that are a complete copy of the mRNA transcribed from the functional gene, those that are only a partial copy of the corresponding mRNA, and those that contain sequences in addition to those expected to be present in the mRNA).

>HEALTHY-6_vial.58097.1gene=HEALTHY-6_vial.58097reference_id=ENST00 000440030ref_gene_id=ENSG00000235559ref_gene_name=NOL5BPcov=5.446237FP KM=0.956689 TPM=0.922521

TGTGAGGAGACGATTGAAAAACCCAAAAAGAAGAAAAAGCAAAAGCCCCA
GGAGATTCATCAGGAGAATGGAATGGAAGACCCATCTATCTCTTTCTCCAAA
CCCAAGAAAAAGAAATCTTTTTCCAAGGAGGAGTTGATGAGTAGCGATCTT
GAAGAGACCGCTGGCAGCACCAGTCTTCCCAAGAGGAAGAAGTCTTCACCC
AAGGAGGAAACAGTTAATGACACCGAAGAGTCAGGCCACAGAAGTGGCTCC
AAGAAAACGAGGAAATTCTCCAAAGAGGAGCTGGTCAGCAGTGGGCCTGAA
GAGGCGGCTGGCAAGAGCAGCTCCAAGAAGAAGAAAAAGTTCCATAAAGC
ATCCCAGGAAGATTAG

>PREDIABETIC.49293.1gene=PREDIABETIC.49293reference_id=ENST000004 40030

ref_gene_id=ENSG00000235559ref_gene_name=NOL5BPcov=6.821105FPKM=1 .281202TPM=0.855955

TGTGAGGAGACGATTGAAAAACCCAAAAAGAAGAAAAAGCAAAAGCCCCA
GGAGATTCATCAGGAGAATGGAATGGAAGACCCATCTATCTCTTTCTCCAAA
CCCAAGAAAAAGAAATCTTTTTCCAAGGAGGAGTTGATGAGTAGCGATCTT
GAAGAGACCGCTGGCAGCACCAGTCTTCCCAAGAGGAAGAAGTCTTCACCC
AAGGAGGAAACAGTTAATGACACCGAAGAGTCAGGCCACAGAAGTGGCTCC

AAGAAAACGAGGAAATTCTCCAAAGAGGAGCTGGTCAGCAGTGGGCCTGAA
GAGGCGGCTGGCAAGAGCAGCTCCAAGAAGAAGAAAAAGTTCCATAAAGC
ATCCCAGGAAGATTAG

In Diabetic Subject (DIABETIC) above Gene name NOL5BP Neucleoprotein Pseudogene not found, not expressed.

c) Location 20 chromosome Upregulated (Protein coding:- Q9BX67 Junctional adhesion molecule C)

>HEALTHY-6_vial.151482.1gene=HEALTHY-6_vial.151482reference_id=ENST 00000570096ref_gene_id=ENSG00000261431ref_gene_name=RP4-616B8.4cov=5.401 070FPKM=0.948755 TPM=0.914870

CTTGAGCGTGGAGGGTAGATGCTTCAGGTGACCTTTTACGAGCGTGGCGTGT
CCTGGATGGCGGCCGCACACTTAGGAAGAACGGGCTTTGGGAGAGGACCGC
TGGCCCGAGAGTGGAACCTTGCACGCACTGGGCGTTGAAGCAGTGCTTTCTG
GATTAAATACGAAATACTGATGTCACAAGCTA

>PREDIABETIC.127702.1gene=PREDIABETIC.127702reference_id=ENST0000 0570096

ref_gene_id=ENSG00000261431ref_gene_name=RP4-616B8.4cov=5.316927FPK M=0.998674TPM=0.667202

CTTGAGCGTGGAGGGTAGATGCTTCAGGTGACCTTTTACGAGCGTGGCGTGT
CCTGGATGGCGGCCGCACACTTAGGAAGAACGGGCTTTGGGAGAGGACCGC
TGGCCCGAGAGTGGAACCTTGCACGCACTGGGCGTTGAAGCAGTGCTTTCTG
GATTAAATACGAAATACTGATGTCACAAGCTA

Not expressed in DIABETIC

d) Location on Chromosome 6 no function (Processed Pseudogenes)

>HEALTHY-6_vial.58787.1gene=HEALTHY-6_vial.58787reference_id=ENST00 000408816ref_gene_id=ENSG00000221743ref_gene_name=Z95152.1   cov=0.668132 FPKM=0.117364 TPM=0.113173

GGTCCTCATTCAAATGCACATTCTAAGGTCTCAACTGCAGACCTGCTGAGTC

ACAAGCCCTG GGGTGGGGCCCAGGAATCTGCATTTTAAC

>PREDIABETIC.49843.1gene=PREDIABETIC.49843reference_id=ENST000004
08816

ref_gene_id=ENSG00000221743ref_gene_name=Z95152.1cov=3.887006FPKM=0
.730093TPM=0.487766

GGTCCTCATTCAAATGCACATTCTAAGGTCTCAACTGCAGACCTGCTGAGTC
ACAAGCCCTG GGGTGGGGCCCAGGAATCTGCATTTTAAC

No expression in diabetic
Gene name ATAD3A Upregulated chromosome 1 (ATpase family Domain AAA)
HEALTHY:-
>HEALTHY-6_vial.143.5gene=HEALTHY-6_vial.143reference_id=ENST00000
439513ref_gene_id=ENSG00000197785ref_gene_name=ATAD3Acov=4.469269FPK
M=0.785075 TPM=0.757035

GGTGTCCGGCCTCCCTCCCGGGGGGCCTTCGCGGGCTTCTGCTGGTGCTTCT
GTGCCTGTGGGTCTGGATTCCTCCAGGGCCTGATCCTGGGTGCAGATGCGGC
TGGAAGCCCTGAGCCTGCTGCACACACTAGTCTGGGCATGGAGTCTCTGCCG
TGCCGGAGCCGTGCAGACACAGGAGCGGCTGTCAGGCAGTGCCAGCCCTGA
GCAAGTGCCAGCTGGTGAGTGCTGTGCTCTGCAGGAGTATGAGGCCGCCGT
GGAGCAGCTCAAGAGCGAGCAGATCCGGGCGCAGGCTGAGGAGAGGAGGA
AGACCCTGAGCGAGGAGACCCGGCAGCACCAGGCCAGGGCCCAGTATCAAG
ACAAGCTGGCCCGGCAGCGCTACGAGGACCAACTGAAGCAGCAG

prediabetic:-

>PREDIABETIC.98.1 gene=PREDIABETIC.98 reference_id=ENST00000439513

ref_gene_id=ENSG00000197785ref_gene_name=ATAD3Acov=0.159636FPKM=
0.029984TPM=0.020032

GGTGTCCGGCCTCCCTCCCGGGGGGCCTTCGCGGGCTTCTGCTGGTGCTTCT
GTGCCTGTGGGTCTGGATTCCTCCAGGGCCTGATCCTGGGTGCAGATGCGGC
TGGAAGCCCTGAGCCTGCTGCACACACTAGTCTGGGCATGGAGTCTCTGCCG
TGCCGGAGCCGTGCAGACACAGGAGCGGCTGTCAGGCAGTGCCAGCCCTGA

GCAAGTGCCAGCTGGTGAGTGCTGTGCTCTGCAGGAGTATGAGGCCGCCGT
GGAGCAGCTCAAGAGCGAGCAGATCCGGGCGCAGGCTGAGGAGAGGAGGA
AGACCCTGAGCGAGGAGACCCGGCAGCACCAGGCCAGGGCCCAGTATCAAG
ACAAGCTGGCCCGGCAGCGCTACGAGGACCAACTGAAGCAGCAG

diabetic:-

>DIABETIC.60.1 gene=DIABETIC.60 reference_id=ENST00000439513

ref_gene_id=ENSG00000197785ref_gene_name=ATAD3Acov=0.474773FPKM=
0.066528TPM=0.050385

GGTGTCCGGCCTCCCTCCCGGGGGGGCCTTCGCGGGCTTCTGCTGGTGCTTCT
GTGCCTGTGGGTCTGGATTCCTCCAGGGCCTGATCCTGGGTGCAGATGCGGC
TGGAAGCCCTGAGCCTGCTGCACACACTAGTCTGGGCATGGAGTCTCTGCCG
TGCCGGAGCCGTGCAGACACAGGAGCGGCTGTCAGGCAGTGCCAGCCCTGA
GCAAGTGCCAGCTGGTGAGTGCTGTGCTCTGCAGGAGTATGAGGCCGCCGT
GGAGCAGCTCAAGAGCGAGCAGATCCGGGCGCAGGCTGAGGAGAGGAGGA
AGACCCTGAGCGAGGAGACCCGGCAGCACCAGGCCAGGGCCCAGTATCAAG
ACAAGCTGGCCCGGCAGCGCTACGAGGACCAACTGAAGCAGCAG

a)   >DIABETIC.14871.2gene=DIABETIC.14871reference_id=ENST0000059
3589 ref_gene_id=ENSG00000230291 ref_gene_name=RP11-244J10.1 cov=0.221219
FPKM=0.030998TPM=0.023477

ATGAAGTTTAATCCCTTTGTGACTTCCGACCGAAGCAAGAATCGCAAAAGGC
ATTTCAACGCACCTTCCCACATTCGAAGGAAGATTATGTCTTCCCTTCTTTCC
AAAGAGCTGAGACAGAAGTACAACGAGCGATCCATGCCCATCCGAAAGGAC
GATGAAGTTCAGGTTGTACGAGGACACTACGAAGGTCAGCAAATTGGCAAA
GTGGTCCAGGTTTACAGGAAGAAATATGTTATCTACATTGAATGGGTGCAGC
GGGAAAAGGCTAATGGCACAACTGTCCACATAGGCATTCACTCCAGCAAGG
TGGTTATCACTAGGCTAAAACTGGACAAAGACAGCAAAAAGATCCTTGAAC
GGAAAGCCAAATCTCGCCAAGTAGGAAAGGAAAAGGGCAAATACAAGGAA
GAAACAATTAGAAG ATGGAGGAATAA

>HEALTHY-6_vial.108899.2gene=HEALTHY-6_vial.108899reference_id=ENS
T00000593589ref_gene_id=ENSG00000230291ref_gene_name=RP11-244J10.1cov=
0.216116 FPKM=0.037963TPM=0.036607

ATGAAGTTTAATCCCTTTGTGACTTCCGACCGAAGCAAGAATCGCAAAAGGC
ATTTCAACGCACCTTCCCACATTCGAAGGAAGATTATGTCTTCCCTTCTTTCC
AAAGAGCTGAGACAGAAGTACAACGAGCGATCCATGCCCATCCGAAAGGAC
GATGAAGTTCAGGTTGTACGAGGACACTACGAAGGTCAGCAAATTGGCAAA
GTGGTCCAGGTTTACAGGAAGAAATATGTTATCTACATTGAATGGGTGCAGC
GGGAAAAGGCTAATGGCACAACTGTCCACATAGGCATTCACTCCAGCAAGG
TGGTTATCACTAGGCTAAAACTGGACAAAGACAGCAAAAAGATCCTTGAAC
GGAAAGCCAAATCTCGCCAAGTAGGAAAGGAAAAGGGCAAATACAAGGAA
GAAACAATTGAGAA GATGGAGGAATAA

b) NOL5BP nucleoprotein Gene has been found expressed in HEALTHY and PREDIABETIC but notin Diabetes.

>HEALTHY-6_vial.58097.1gene=HEALTHY-6_vial.58097reference_id=ENST00
000440030ref_gene_id=ENSG00000235559 ref_gene_name=NOL5BP cov=5.446237
FPKM=0.956689 TPM=0.922521

TGTGAGGAGACGATTGAAAAACCCAAAAAGAAGAAAAAGCAAAAGCCCCA
GGAGATTCATCAGGAGAATGGAATGGAAGACCCATCTATCTCTTTCTCCAAA
CCCAAGAAAAAGAAATCTTTTTCCAAGGAGGAGTTGATGAGTAGCGATCTT
GAAGAGACCGCTGGCAGCACCAGTCTTCCCAAGAGGAAGAAGTCTTCACCC
AAGGAGGAAACAGTTAATGACACCGAAGAGTCAGGCCACAGAAGTGGCTCC
AAGAAAACGAGGAAATTCTCCAAAGAGGAGCTGGTCAGCAGTGGGCCTGAA
GAGGCGGCTGGCAAGAGCAGCTCCAAGAAGAAGAAAAAGTTCCATAAAGC
ATCCCAGGAAGATTAG

>PREDIABETIC.49293.1gene=PREDIABETIC.49293reference_id=ENST000004
40030

ref_gene_id=ENSG00000235559ref_gene_name=NOL5BPcov=6.821105FPKM=1
.281202TPM=0.855955

TGTGAGGAGACGATTGAAAAACCCAAAAAGAAGAAAAAGCAAAAGCCCCA
GGAGATTCATCAGGAGAATGGAATGGAAGACCCATCTATCTCTTTCTCCAAA
CCCAAGAAAAAGAAATCTTTTTCCAAGGAGGAGTTGATGAGTAGCGATCTT
GAAGAGACCGCTGGCAGCACCAGTCTTCCCAAGAGGAAGAAGTCTTCACCC
AAGGAGGAAACAGTTAATGACACCGAAGAGTCAGGCCACAGAAGTGGCTCC
AAGAAAACGAGGAAATTCTCCAAAGAGGAGCTGGTCAGCAGTGGGCCTGAA

GAGGCGGCTGGCAAGAGCAGCTCCAAGAAGAAGAAAAAGTTCCATAAAGC
ATCCCAGGAAGATTAG

In Diabetic Subject above Gene name NOL5BP Neucleoprotein Pseudogene not found, not expressed.

c)Located on chromosome 12 Downregulated (ribosomal protein)

>HEALTHY-6_vial.106140.1gene=HEALTHY-6_vial.106140reference_id=ENST
00000495623ref_gene_id=ENSG00000243517ref_gene_name=RP11-627K11.1cov=4.4
44179 FPKM=0.780667TPM=0.752785

GGCAGAGGTGCAGGTCCTGGTGCTTGATGGTCGAGGCCATCTCCTGGGCCGC
CTGGCGGCCATCGTGGTAAACAGGTACTGCTGGGCCGGAAGGTGGTGGTCGT
ACGCTGCGAAGGCATCAACATTTCTGGCAATTTCTACAGAAACAAGTTGAAG
TACCTCGCTTTCCTCCGCAAGCGGATGAACACCAACTCTTACCGAGGCTCCT
ACCACTTCCGGGCCCCCAGCCGCATCTTCTGGCGGACCGTGCGAGGTATGCT
GCCCCACAAGACCAAGCGAGGCCAGGCCGCTCTGGACCGCCTCAAGGTGTT
TGATGGCATCCCACCGCCCTACGACAAGAAAAAGCGGATGGTGGTTCCTGTT
GCCCTCAAGGTTGTGCGTCTGAAGCCTACAAGAAAGTTTGCCTATCTGGGGC
GCCTGGCTCACGAGTTTGGCTGGAAGTACCAGGCAGGGACAGCCACCCTGG
AGGAGAAGAGGAAAGAGAAAGCCAAGATCCACTACGGGAAGAAGAAACAG
CTCATGAGGCTACGGAAACAGGCCGAGAAGAACGTGGAGAAGAAAATTGA
CAAATACACAGAGGTCCTCAAGACCCACGGCCTCCTG ATC

>PREDIABETIC.90093.1gene=PREDIABETIC.90093reference_id=ENST000004
95623

ref_gene_id=ENSG00000243517ref_gene_name=RP11-627K11.1cov=2.192012FP
KM=0.411724TPM=0.275068

GGCAGAGGTGCAGGTCCTGGTGCTTGATGGTCGAGGCCATCTCCTGGGCCGC
CTGGCGGCCATCGTGGTAAACAGGTACTGCTGGGCCGGAAGGTGGTGGTCG
TACGCTGCGAAGGCATCAACATTTCTGGCAATTTCTACAGAAACAAGTTGAA
GTACCTCGCTTTCCTCCGCAAGCGGATGAACACCAACTCTTACCGAGGCTCC
TACCACTTCCGGGCCCCCAGCCGCATCTTCTGGCGGACCGTGCGAGGTATGC
TGCCCCACAAGACCAAGCGAGGCCAGGCCGCTCTGGACCGCCTCAAGGTGT
TTGATGGCATCCCACCGCCCTACGACAAGAAAAAGCGGATGGTGGTTCCTGT

TGCCCTCAAGGTTGTGCGTCTGAAGCCTACAAGAAAGTTTGCCTATCTGGGG
CGCCTGGCTCACGAGTTTGGCTGGAAGTACCAGGCAGGGACAGCCACCCTG
GAGGAGAAGAGGAAAGAGAAAGCCAAGATCCACTACGGGAAGAAGAAACA
GCTCATGAGGCTACGGAAACAGGCCGAGAAGAACGTGGAGAAGAAAATTG
ACAAATACACAGAGGTCCTCAAGACCCACGGCCTCCTGATC

>DIABETIC.14437.1 gene=DIABETIC.14437 reference_id=ENST00000495623

ref_gene_id=ENSG00000243517ref_gene_name=RP11-627K11.1cov=2.050880
FPKM=0.287380TPM=0.217647

GGCAGAGGTGCAGGTCCTGGTGCTTGATGGTCGAGGCCATCTCCTGGGCCGC
CTGGCGGCCATCGTGGTAAACAGGTACTGCTGGGCCGGAAGGTGGTGGTCGT
ACGCTGCGAAGGCATCAACATTTCTGGCAATTTCTACAGAAACAAGTTGAAG
TACCTCGCTTTCCTCCGCAAGCGGATGAACACCAACTCTTACCGAGGCTCCT
ACCACTTCCGGGCCCCCAGCCGCATCTTCTGGCGGACCGTGCGAGGTATGCT
GCCCCACAAGACCAAGCGAGGCCAGGCCGCTCTGGACCGCCTCAAGGTGTT
TGATGGCATCCCACCGCCCTACGACAAGAAAAAGCGGATGGTGGTTCCTGTT
GCCCTCAAGGTTGTGCGTCTGAAGCCTACAAGAAAGTTTGCCTATCTGGGGC
GCCTGGCTCACGAGTTTGGCTGGAAGTACCAGGCAGGGACAGCCACCCTGG
AGGAGAAGAGGAAAGAGAAAGCCAAGATCCACTACGGGAAGAAGAAACAG
CTCATGAGGCTACGGAAACAGGCCGAGAAGAACGTGGAGAAGAAAATTGAC
AAATACACAGAGGTCCTCAAGACCCACGGCCTCCTGATC

Above mentioned fasta sequences from a) to h) are some examples of gene transcripts which are utilized in metabolic pathways, cellular processes and in gene ontology are shortlisted based on there log FC2 value working on UP and DOWN regulated are studied, where some of them are found to be expressed in healthy while prediabetic and diabetic are found to be pseudogenes or some of them found altered/ mutated with SNPs (single nucleotide polymorphism) while most of the transcript in diabetic are not expressed, which indicates the hormonal (ligand) disturbed binding process, which doesn't able to activate receptors, when then doesn't regulated intracellular metabolic events, which lead to alteration and mismatch of the fragments that shows the effect of Diabetic in the subject and alteration of the genomic sequence and disturbance in gene ontology is observed in the studied sample.

Chapter VI. Discussion

My study basically is an cross sectional observational study where analysis is done to study the functions of genes involved in Type 2 Diabetes Mellitus, Prediabetic, and healthy subjects. The aim of the present research work was to analyze differential gene Expression / Gene clusters involved in central dogma, attributable to Type II Diabetes Mellitus from the Biological Databases and to stretch the analysis further with whole transcriptome (WTA) in samples.

In this study a well defined pateints with and without Type 2 diabetes Mellitus has been studied. The samples were collected based on ADA (American Diabetic Association) 2016 criterio for Diabetic Mellitus and Prediabetic and proceeded for Transcriptome Analysis [Table no 4]. samples has been extracted and has been transported to Xcelris Ltd, Ahmedabad for Exome Sequencing.

We analysed the purity of RNA extracting with Trizol Method [290] where target was to isolate pureform of mRNA in studied sample which gives the idea of differential expresssed genes and coding region, to separate mRNA from rRNA and tRNA, mRNA as been enriched by implementing poly A tailing attachment process, Poly A tail will help to make mRNA in circular form which will help to replicate and amplify the RNA for further processing of developing the cDNA library that is called as mRNA enrichment. RNA purity concentration ratio at A260/280 was obtained in healthy is 2.01, prediabetic is 1.89 and diabetic is 1.97, with standard values it indicates the purity in RNA should be 2.0 which has been obtained in Healthy sample, whereas some probable contaminants involved in Prediabetic and Diabetic sample. Present study are similar to previous studies done (292) where concentration has been checked by using MALDI TOF mass Spectrometer Jong Wong Choi Et al 2017 (283), whereas studied samples purity, concentration and yield at A260/280 angstrom are performed by Nanodrop 8000 spectrophotometer. Also quality checked of total RNA (28S, 18S and 5S) which indicates the large and small subunit in the studied sample, where healthy shows the clear band of large and small subunits, comparatively prediabetic and diabetic sample showed light band which indicates some abnormal morphology noted on 1% formaldehyde Gel Electrophoresis (figure7) similar kind of study was undertaken by chandrakumar satishkumar et al 2018 (280) have checked the rna quality at nanodrop 2000 spectrophotometer.

Mean Size of the library profile of the studied sample were extracted by using 2 X

150 BP end onIllumina Platform (figure 10), where we obtained mean of healthy sample is 302 BP, prediabetic is 299 and diabetic is also found 299 BP (basepairs) which indicates the equal number of concentrations, by which the value of each sequencing run increased the number of samples that can be sequenced in asingle run, unequal concetnration may lead to biased representation of certain libraries over others. Based on the illumina platform prepared cDNA, high quality sequence data (healthy-7,842,978,223 bp, prediabetic-7,391,654,813 bp and diabetic-8,233,839,132 BP) (Table 6) has been generated. Those obtained sequences are then mapped with reference genome GrCh37.P13 (The reference genome ofHuman (GRCh37.p13, genome size ~ 3.2Gb) and the corresponding GTF file was downloaded from Ensembl database (https://grch37.ensembl.org/Homo_sapie ns/Info/Annotation#assembly)). (Table 7,8). And mapped reads are observed in healthy (42711396), Prediabetic (40816672), Diabetic (54534553)using HISAT2 (Heirarchical Indexing for Spliced alignment of Transcripts) software.which was not reported in any previous study taking human subject, some authors Oliver Kluth, Daniel Matzkeet al 2014 (281) studied the same transcriptome sequencing on mouse islet diabetes susceptibility genes. We further merged the transcripts by Stringtie, a consensus set of transcripts are obtained in BAM(Binary alignment Map) format by Stringtie Merger of all the gene structure in studied sample.FPKMvalue and Log 2 FC value generated (Figure 9, 10) for Differential Gene Expression (DEG) where coding regions, pseudogenes and gene transcripts genomic elements are observed (Table no 8).

Analysis started with mapping reads of all samples individually against the *Homo sapiens* (GRCh37.p13) reference genome to identify the positions from where the reads originated. This mapping information allows us to collect subsets of the reads corresponding to each gene, and then to assemble and quantify transcripts represented by those reads. Hence the high quality reads were mapped to *Human* genome using **HISAT2** (Heirarchical Indexing for Spliced alignment of transcripts) to create alignment in BAM (Binary alignment Map) format for each sample. First step is indexing the reference genome using hisat-build (HISAT2 specific indexer program). Then the input reads, in FASTQ format, were given to HISAT2 aligner along with the reference genome index and create splice-site aware alignments individually for all 3 samples (Table 9).

In our RNA-seq experiment, it is crucial to have accurate reconstructions of all the isoforms expressed from each gene, as well as estimates of the relative abundance of those isoforms. **StringTie** assembles transcripts from RNA-seq reaDiabetic that have been aligned to the genome, first grouping the reaDiabetic into distinct gene loci and then

149

assembling each locus into as many isoforms as are needed to explain the data. Following this, StringTie simultaneously assembles and quantify the final transcripts by using network flow algorithm and starting from most highly abundant transcripts. The GTF annotation files, containing exon-intron structures of "known" genes, are then used to annotate the assembled transcripts and quantify the expression of known genes as well derive clues if a novel transcript has been found in the studied sample (Table 10, Graph 3). After assembling each sample, the full set of assemblies is passed to StringTie's merge function, which merges together all the gene structures found in any of the samples. This step is required because transcripts in some of the samples might only be partially covered by reads, and as a consequence only partial versions of them will be assembled in the initial StringTie run.

The output consists of assembled gene/transcript GTF file for all samples. The merging step produced 3,17,407 transcripts in the form of a GTF file. The extracted transcript sequences (using gff read program) of all 3 samples in fasta format along with the corresponding GTF files are constructed.

Differential Expressed Genes (DEG):- After Mapping between refference genome and transcripts of the studied samples is mapped, FPKM (Fragment per kilobase per million reads mapped) and Log 2 FC value (transform value) (Figure 9,10) were extracted to raw counts of each genes. Those obtained value will decide the UP and DOWN Stream process of the reads (Table 11). Statistics application carried out in these regards of T2DM, revealed that less number of genes in UP and more in DOWN regulations are observed, contrary to the observation in Healthy and Prediaebetic , where reverse of the observation these observations is noted.

Apart from UP and DOWN regulation gene numbers in healthy, prediabetic and diabetic, top 50 genes based on LOG2FC value (Table 13) (25 UP regulated and 25 DOWN regulated) has been shortlisted to know the chromosomal locations, functions and there expression variants. Those 50 genes has been graphically represented in Heatmap using R software which shows the color coding regions from Red, Green and Yellow, indicating lowly expressed, moderate expressed and highly expressed, we observed most of the genes up and down regulated in diabetic are in red color which is low expression of genes, whereas in prediabetic most of the genes in Red and Some are observed Yellow in Color indicating Low and Moderate Gene Expression, contrary in healthy most of the genes are in Yellow and very few are observed Green in color, expressing moderate and High Gene Expression.

150

These observation of UP and DOWN regulation FPKM value based are in diabetic, prediabetic and healthy are unique in the sense as regards. values are unique in the study and not reported by other researcher. Heat map color Graphical representation also undertaken and analysed in our study for noticing/ revealing heavy, moderate and mild fluctuations in UP and DOWN regulations (figure 11).

The study is stretched to analyse top 50 genes (25 UP and 25 DOWN regualted genes) basedon FPKM (Fragment per kilobase per million reads mapped) value selected for analysing the P-Value (tounderstand the statistical significance when it is very unlikely to have occurred given the Null or alternative hypothesis), Mean, and Standard deviation to understand the normal distribution between the shortlisted datasets in healthy, prediabetic and diabetic, equal or unequal distribution in UP regulation and DOWN regulation stream is carried out, we analysed, Shapiro Wilk Test for nrmality of the dataset, Mean and SD was calculated by using Kruskal-Wallis Test (Table 6 & 7), and comparison of those means obtained between groups and Chi-square values have been calculated by Mann-Whitney U Test, which signifies unequal distibution of the data set between the groups, (table 22) also mean value in top 25 upregualted genes are observed drastically variants, which indicates the mutational behavior in UP regualtion process, as gene expression effecting the down regulation process for transcriptional and translational elements. Which further effects the metabolism process of the cell and its components. Same process of normality by Shapiro –wilk test, mean, SD and P-value by Kruskal Wallis test and comparison of mean by Mann Whitney U test was applied top 25 genes in DOWN regualtion process shortlisted by FPKM value, we observed the unequal distribution in the data sets which indicates the mutational effect on DOWN regulation as genes are not expressed or over expressed in UP regualtion definitely it effects on DOWN regulation processed for mRNA (transcription) and protein (Translation) development process (graph 12), on comparative analysis of UP and DOWN regulation mean value (table 25) indicates healthy, showing apropriate value in both, whereas drastic changed value can be observed in prediabetic and diabetic, where UP shows more value compared with DOWN , which shouldbe reversed if there is no hormonal imbalance or mutations. of different sample the FPKM value of top50 genes comparing Healthy, Prediabetic and Diabetic subject showing the Differential expression Genes, their location of chromosomes, gene ID from database, we further observed and analysed highlighting Ubiquinine, one of the key factor for ATP, NADH energy generator in Electron Transport Chain located on chromosome 7, 20, 6, there Transformed fold value obtained is fluctuating in prediabetic and diabetic which indicates the functionality of the gene and there expression level low is observed in prediabetic and diabetic, and moderate expression in healthy.

151

Further differential Genes exclusively expressed in healthy 48552, prediabetic 1993, anddiabetic 946 (table 15, graph 4), graphically those number are bifurcated in up and down regulations in healthy vs prediabetic (table 16), and healthy vs diabetic (table 18). (table 22, 24) statistically overall expression of all the genes in different compared categories are healthy=6444, prediabetic= 2193, and diabetic = 2101 are observed, which was not reported by any previous study.

Gene Ontology:- The Gene Ontology provides controlled vocabularies of defined terms representing gene product properties. These cover three domains: **Cellular Component**, the parts of a cell or its extracellular environment; **Molecular Function**, the elemental activities of a gene product at the molecular level, such as binding or catalysis; and **Biological Process**, operations or sets of molecular events with a defined beginning and end, pertinent to the functioning of integrated living units: cells, tissues, organs, and organisms. In our study GO (Gene Ontology) study was performed by uploading Gene ID's on Biomart of Differential Expressed Genes of studied sample viz; Healthy, Prediabetic and Diabetic Sample.

In Biological process (figure 13-15) shows the functions and number of genes involved in the processes like translation, signal transduction, protein transport, gene expression and apoptotic process are few, in comparative to all three samples (healthy, prediabetic and diabetic) overall prediabetic (translation=525, gene expression 530, and apoptotic process=376) showed the less number of gene expression compared with diabetic and healthy, (table 25 and graph 13), which indicates the genetic mutation and expression plays an important role in biological process.

In Cellular Component (figure 16-18) shows the functions and number of genes involved in the cell maintainance like Plasma Membrane, Cytoplasm, Nucleus, mitochondria and Golgi Apparatus, overall in prediabetic gene expression number in said cellular process like plasma membrane =1283, golgi apparatus = 322, nucleus = 3090 are observed and found very less as compared with diabetic and healthy (Table 26, Graph 14).

Another segment is Molecular Functions in GO, which graphically representing (figure 19- 21) the number of genes against the molecular functions like:- DNA, ATP, RNA Binding, Protein kinaseactivity,catalytic activity are observed, overall in prediabetic gene expression are found to be less in every function as compared with healthy and diabetic.

Glucose transport, WNT signaling, muscle development, pancreas development genes, and insulinsignaling pathway were associated with hypermethylation process in subjects with predaibetic and diabetic, although I-kappa B kinase/ NF-kappa B cascade were observed in Prediabetic and diabetic metabolic cycle, associated genes in these pathway were different in each sample. Finding are same reported by previous study reported by Tandi E, Matsha, 2016 (289).

Comparatively of all studied subjects i.e, healthy, prediabetic and diabetic in all categories of Gene Ontology we observed that Prediabetic Subject has shown less Genetic Expression (about 50%) variation has noted compared with diabetic and healthy, which indicates in Gene ontology vocabulary any of the categories is geneticaly modified or mutated by SNP's or Pseudogenes there effect is direct proportionate to other categories.

Pathway Analysis:- In our study ortholog (means any of two or more homologous gene sequence found in different species related to linear descent) and mapping of the transcripts to the biological pathways were performed using KAAS (KEGG Automatic Annotation Server) (table 2 -8).

All the differential expressed genes were compared against the KEGG Database using BLAST X (translated nucleotide to protein) with threshold value of 60.

The mapped transcripts represents metabolic pathways of major biomolecules such as carbohydrates, lipids, nucleotides, amino acids, glycans, co factor, vitamins, trepenoids, polyketoids etc. the mapped genes also represented the number of genes involved in metabolism, genetic information processes, environmental information, and other categories like cellular processes etc (Table 28).

As the study is focused on Type 2 Diabetes Mellitus, in metabolic pathway study we focused on Gycolysis, TCA (kreb's Cycle) and Electron Transport Chain (ETC), there genetic alteration, andenzymatic involvement and there disturbance in the process, while observing the studied samplesmetabolic pathway focusing on glycolysis it has been noted that MAPK1 (mitogen activated protein kinase1) were found expressed in healthy and in diabetic but not observed expressed in prediabetic, Mitogen protein kinase which activates multiple biochemical signals in cellular process such as proliferation, transcription, regulation and development of cell is found effected in prediabetic, compared with healthy and diabetic.

IRS2, (Insulin Receptor Substrate 2) located on chromosome 13 is observed expressed in healthy and diabetic same is not expressed in prediabetic, also IRS4 (Insulin Receptor Substrate 4) has been additionally observed in prediabetic and diabetics, which indicates that in the infectious state additional receptor mechanism is activated also it proves that genetic alteration gives adverse and unwanted effect in cell metabolisms (Table 29-31). Figure (22-24) graphically represents the glycolysis pathway in healthy, prediabetic and diabetic indicating the expression of genes an enzymatic activity in Black (expressed) and Red (not expressed or over expressed) in the pathway, the arrow indicates the molecular interactions between the enzymes, and indirect link or unknown reactions, properand complete gylcolysis has been observed in prediabetic, diabetic compared with healthy, whereenzyme class 3.1.3.1.1 Hydrolase (Fructose Diphosphate) is not expressed in healthy, whereas it is expressed in prediabetic and diabetic showing additional class to activation in the glycolysis, where insulin resistance and no absorption of glucose takes place, also some other fluctuations in the enzymaticclasses in glycolysis in healthy vs prediabetic and healthy vs diabetic has been observed and noted (table 32), this kind of kegg pathway analysis of healthy, prediabetic and diabetic is not reported in literature previously.

Further the study is stretched to observe the genetic and enzymatic variants in studied sample (healthy, prediabetic and diabetic) in TCA (Tricarboxylic Acid Cycle) Kreb's Cycle, one of the cycle occurs in Matrix of Mitochondria where E.C (enzyme Classification) 1.1.1.42 (class oxidoreductase, enzyme isocitrate dehydrogenase is observed in healthy and diabetic and no expression is observed in healthy, arrow indicates molecular interactions between the enzymes and arrow indicates the indirect link or unknown reaction are observed. TCA / Kreb's Cycle reactions are observed with some enzymaticchanges compared healthy with prediabetic and diabetic (figure 25-27). again which indicates thegenetic alteration , mutation and variants in prediabetic is found more as compared with healthy and diabetic.

Also one of the important cycle where free energy released druing the oxidation of glucose to CO2 isretained in the reduced to Co-Enzyme NADH and FADH2, generated during glycolysis and TCA cycle. Electrons are released from NADH and FADH2 and eventually transferred to O2 forming H2O. In KEGG Pathway Diagram including the oxidative Phosphorylation System (OXPHOS) genes selected by trancriptome analysis of healthy, prediabetic and diabetic sample, where (figure 28-30) where in the upper part 6 respiratory chain complex with the corresponding E.C number are observed same in all studied sample, in bottom rectangles are indicating the subunits of each respiratory chain complex, the subunits encoded by genes studied by microarray analysis are shown in black

154

color rectangles. The subunits in the complex III (cytochrome Bc1 Complex) and Complex IV (Cytochrome C Oxidase) has been observed mutated in E/B/A comples in prediabetic sample, whereas found same in healthy and diabetic, also Cytochrome C oxidase complex IV is found not expressed in prediabetic, and found expressed in healthy and diabetic.

Comparative analysis of above mentioned metabolic pathways, Glycolysis, Kreb's Cycle and ETC (electron transport chain) indicates the genetic mutations, alterations where enzymatic variants areobserved more in Prediabetic and Diabetic as compared with Healthy mapped with Reference Genome, which gives the improper functioning of the cell which has been observed more in prediabetic ans diabetic compared with healthy. Chandra shekahr vasamsetty et al 2011 (281) Similar kind of study have been done in recent past based on Diabetic with parental history and without parental history has been found same in current study also, various genes involved in inositol metabolism, starch, sucrose, MAPK signalling pathway, Glycolysis, gluconeogenesis, neurodegenerative disorders etc wereobserved.

Genetic Alteration: - In these study, implementing Bioinformatics and their methods, various tools led to conclude the similarity, structure robustness and there activity in causing disease of Diabetes Mellitus Type II . Q-Mean shows the quality score of the said structures from diabetic to healthy, ranging from -to -2.79 (Table 37), which concludes the quality of the structure between experimental Structure and target database structure, as nearer to Zero (0) (Graph:1) will have optimum and good quality score from the perspective of functionality, mobility and energy level of subjects taken. After performing the Swiss model score generated led to conclude the average quality of the structure as -4.0 or below led to conclude low quality of the structure, which is of no use for further analysis.

Lastly out of 50 top differentially expressed genes, few UP and DOWN regulated genes has been shortlisted based on there locations on chromosomes 6,20,1,7 has been studied for there translation process by developing there ORF (Open Reading Frame) by using ExPASY (Expert Protein Assesment Analysis System) provides 3' to 5' frames and 5' to 3' frames, and Q-Mean of individual sequencesfrom healthy, prediabetic and diabetic have been used to produce 3D structure to check the Qualilty of the molecule and degree of nativeness in the studied structure, where we observed that E-Value (similarity) Q-Mean Degree of Nativeness) in healthy(-1.02) is closer to 1, whereas the Prediabetic (-2.79) and Diabetic (-2.78) are nearer to each other but not closer to degree of nativeness (table 37) . alsoif we closely observe the structure of studied molecules one can observe the absence of loop inprediabetic and diabetic, and can see that loop in healthy , (Table 37) these type of structural assesment highlighting ɑ alpha helix, β sheets , turns (loop) and Quality score check is not reported in any of the previous literature usind 3D visualization and mathematical approach.

Also the results based on FPKM, and SNPs found on the transcriptome data obtained after completing the Whole transcriptome analysis (WTA) (Table 36, 37) , here one nucleic acid G is found mutated in prediabetic sample while t is found same in healthy and diabetic sample, also transcriptome based values of FPKM found more in prediabetic (prediabetic subject) as compare to healthy and diabetic (healthy and Diabetic) subject located on chromosome 12 (Graph 18). In chromosome 12 a fragment of 487 base pairs were found in all subjects out of whom one or two single nucleotide polymorphism is found at the end of that pseudogene (table 36), the gene performs the functions like protein junctional adhesion, also counter as receptor of JAM2, mediating leukocyte platelets interaction also play a role in angiogenesis,which initiates VEGF (vascular enhancer growth factor and its receptor).

Another gene which studied is located on chromosome 6 upregulated comprises of 312 base pairs here the fragment is not found expressed in diabetic whereas it is observed in prediabetic and healthy which is used to perform the function as processed pseudogenes given by Gene Card.

One more gene ATAD3A (Atpase family Domain 3 A) gene is found expressed in all subjects and no polymorphism, and genetic alteration is observed, which is located on chromosome 1 performs to prepare the ribosomal protein complex in the cell maintainence.

These kind of SNPs polymorphism in Chinese populations was reported by Liyuan Han 2016 (292), and some sixty five common variants observed by Mandy, Abbas Deghan 2008 (286), were observed same in the studied samples, also Jong wook Choi etal 2017 (283), showed diabetic and prediabetic genetic study and observed 3 SNPs which showed the prediabetic associated genetic ploymorphism at chromosome 7p15,same kind of the data observed in current study too.

After Whole Transcriptome Analysis (WTA). Which concludes that there are various SNPs involved in human chromosome located on different region, these single nucleotide polymorphism may lead to pseudogenes which will not code for protein in the cell, which lead to incomplete functioning of the body and make more susceptible and prone to various clinical and sub clinical complications. Also thoseSNPs found can play vital role in disturbing the metabolic pathways and can give some complication and metabolic disorders.

Several traits like obesity, insulin resistance and increased levels of pro inflammatory cytokines precede and accompany T2DM. On the other hand, it is widely accepted that T2DM has a hereditary component. Hence, it is natural to expect patients suffering from hereditarily transferred predisposition to T2DM to have one or more SNPs/Pseudogenes,mutations are responsible for accelerated progression of underlying traits.

Technical revolution in the field of genetics has allowed identification of numerous genetic variants that associate with T2D. The genetic landscape of T2D susceptibility is as yet incomplete, thus far only explaining a small proportion of the total heritability of diabetes. Many possibilities to dissectthe architecture of T2D etiology have emerged in the form of large-scale genetic studies, meta analyses and sequencing in families. If has already greatly contributed to our understanding of disease mechanisms by identifying pathways that could not be linked to diabetes by existing hypothetical models, even though many genetic findings are very recent and have yet to make their contribution to our knowledge about diabetes pathogenesis. However, one must bear in mind that diabetes is probably a much more diverse disease than the current subdivision into T2D implies and more precise subdivision into subgroups may both facilitate the investigation of T2D genetics and pave the way of more indivdualized treatment.

Typically, SNPs have been used as markers to search for the real determinant of a disease in linkage disequilibria with it. As previously mentioned, the use of functional SNPs, which may be the real disease determinants, could be an important factor in increasing the sensitivity of association tests.

Despite the obvious importance that alterations in the regulation, expression level or splicing of genes can have for the phenotype, these have long been ignored in the most common approaches to finding functional SNPs, which have instead focused more on the possible effect of polymorphisms causing amino acid changes.

After adopting modifiable risk factors, to make watch on Pre diabetic patients to control to convert into healthy and not moving towards diabetic one. One more aspect can be implemented in future about to correlate the method for functional finding in the sequences. Also to target the SNPs and Pseudogene involved in it. Here in this work target to highlight the genetic variation in metabolic pathway too, where fructose diphospate found off (not expressed) EC- 3.1.1.11 in prediabetic and diabetic compared with healthy subject.

Based on these scientific finding, genetic factor is not the only determinant, the interaction of environmental and genetic factors, and the degree to which they interact, should not be underestimated regarding disease development.

The multifaceted approaches to understanding this complex disease together with cheap and fast genotyping as well as developmentof novel genetic statistical tools already helped and will keep leading us to define further the complicated web of genetic and environmental factors contributing to T2DM pathogenesis. It is important to realise that as the roles that dietary and lifestyle choice plays in this complex disease are understood better and better, genetics therapy alone is not sufficient to target the complex disease effectively. Therefore, personalised life style management and genetic therapies should be applied to T2DM patients simultaneously. These combined efforts will speed up molecular genetics driven developments of antidiabetic therapeutics and diabetes prevention.

Chapter VII. Conclusion

✓ The present study was undertaken for Gene expression analysis using Bioinformatics, Data mining in Diabetic, Prediabetic and compared with healthy subject sample, studies are abundant in diabetic comparing with healthy using Genome Wide Association Studies (GWAS) however prediabetic sample studies are finger countable.

✓ In the present study Quantification of the sample for yield purity for RNA is undertaken by 1% formaldehyde agarose gel (figure no 9), and absorption spectra of the samples were tested using Nanodrop 8000 spectrophotometer, we avoided use of MALDI TOF method as present analysis is based on nano level with high defined accuracy.

✓ In the present analysis we observed total number of genes in Healthy found 6091, Prediabetic is 1992, and Diabetic is 946 study further stretched to analyzed to Up and Down Regulation in cell maintainance (Table 12, graph 04).

✓ Up and Down regulation was studied implementing FPKM value (which is Log2 FC calculation (Figure 9, 10, Table 11) which gave top 50 genes in healthy, prediabetic and diabetic representing Up and Down regulation respectively (Graph 5,6,7) the present study with FPKM further advanced method which differs from TPM used in recent past to these present FPKM which analyses fragment per kilobases per molecule and provides the accurate expression value.

✓ While analysing Gene ontology in the present study we observed, Cellular Component reduced much in prediabetic as compared to diabetic in comparison to normal phenomenon in healthy, other component of gene ontology viz: Molecular function, Biological process also have shown similar type of observational findings.(Table 25-27, Figure, 13-21, Graph 13-15)

✓ WE observed in the present study genes involved in metabolic pathways like glycolysis, Tricarboxylic cycle, Ribosome structure, androgen, estrogen metabolism, MAPK signalling pathway, vitamins cofactor are upregulated where as phenylalanine, tyrosine, PPARG are downregulated which ought to have been upregulated as in healthy subject these observation could be linked to number of differentially expressed genes observed in prediabetic (1992) and diabetic (946). (table 27, graph 15).

✓ While analyzing Single nucleotide polymorphism (SNPs) and pseudogenes we recognised one nucleic acid G (Guanine) is found mutated in prediabetic sample while t (thyamine) is found same in healthy and diabetic sample,(Table 3) these reveals the single nucleotide mutation responsible for the abnormalities of prediabetes distinctly different from diabetes.

✓ As regarDiabetic appearance of pseudogenes in the present study we notice 5SNPs (Pseudogenes- genes which are not coding protein) we observed on chormosome 20, 6 and 1 having genes which are not expressed in the transciptome sequencing; revealing that in diabetic upregualtion on said chromosomes are defective. (not producing protiens). (Table 33-37).

✓ Those obtained SNPs may lead to alter the protein structure (Q-Mean) ORF (open Reading Frames) which are utilised in various metabolism processes are found structural altered, where onecan observe the complete loop (blue, cyan color) (table 38, graph 18) is observed missing in Prediabetic and diabetic sample. Specific color indicates the specific amino acid in the 3D structure, where cyan color indicates glutamine and aspargine is altered in prediabetic,and in diabetic compared with healthy in expasy server.

Future Recommendations

✓ Further epigenetics analysis may help if undertaken from the sample healthy/prediabetic and diabetic one can predict the diabetic development/ occurance in pedigree with on isolation in them however this would require Micro RNA analysis in them. Presently to study Micro RNA one has to spent approximately 75,000/- INR Per Sample.

✓ The study can be further interlinked to pharmacokinetics, pharmacogenetics, development ofenzyme substrate complex in newer medicine affecting abnormal pathways.

✓ With the help of these study customised genomic panel can be used to isolate the affecting genes in Diabetes Mellitus, and correlation in there metabolic pathway by reversing the pathway chances of healthy gene expression can be observed.

Drawbacks of the present study

The present study is not based on analysing the complete genome, it focuses chiefly on transcripts and Genome Wide Association Study (GWAs) for analysing Differential Expressed Genes (DEG) in Healthy, Prediabetic and Diabetic Subject, it lacks the information of introns hence we suggest future aspects can be undertaken are :-

1) Epigenetic study of Micro RNA study which are equally important in the genomics of DiabetesMellitus.

160

2) If micro RNA study undertaken the study of the role of the genome in drug response.(Pharmacogenomics).

Chapter VII Bibliography

1. Unwin N, etal "The IDF Diabetes atlas; providing evidence, raising awareness and promoting action". Diabets Res Clin Pract.2010;8(7):2-3.
2. International Diabetes Federation (IDF) Diabetes Atlas,IDF Executive office.2011;5:17-19.
3. Groop L, Et al, "Genetics of Type 2 Diabetes. An overview". Endocrinal Nutr.2009;56:34-37.
4. Stankov K, et al, Genetics and epigenetics factors in etiology of Diabetes Mellitus type I. pediatric 2013;13(2):1112-1123.
5. Mortazavi A, Williams BA, McCue K, Schaeffer L, Wold B: Mapping and quantifying mammalian transcriptomes by RNA-Seq. Nat Methods 2008;5(7):621-628.
6. Chen G, Wang C, Shi T: Overview of available methoDiabetic for diverse RNA-Seq data analyses.Sci China Life Sci. 2011;5(4):1121-1128.
7. Oshlack A, Robinson MD, Young MD: From RNA-seq reaDiabetic to differential expressionresults. Genome Biol.2010;1(3):211- 220.
8. Agarwal A, Koppstein D, Rozowsky J, S boner A, Habegger L, Hillier LW, Sasidharan R, Reinke V, Waterston RH, Gerstein M: Comparison and calibration of transcriptome data from RNA-Seq and tiling arrays. BMC Genomics 2010;1(4):375-383.
9. Bradford JR, Hey Y, Yates T, Li Y, Pepper SD, Miller CJ: A comparison of massively parallel nucleotide sequencing with oligonucleotide microarrays for global transcription profiling. BMC Genomics 2010;11(5):275-282.
10. Immamura M, Et al, Genetics of type 2 diabetes: the era and future perspectives"Endocrinology Journal.2011;58(9):723-39.
11. Talib et al, Study of genome wide association (GWAS) to analyze SNPs and Psuedogenes in Type 2 Diabetes Mellitus, Research Journal of Life Science, Bioinformatics, Pharmaceutical and Chemical Sciences (RJLBPCS).2018;4(5):434-442.
12. G Stoesser, W.Baker, and Et al The EMBL nucleotide sequence database. Nucleic Acids Res. 2002;30(1):21-26.
13. Y Tateno, S.Miyakazi and Et al, DNA Databank of Japan (DDBJ) for genome scale research inlife science. Nucleic Acids Res.2002;30(1):27-30.
14. M D Adams, JM Kelley, and Et al, Complementary DNA Sequencing: expressed sequence tags and human genome project. Science.2013;25(2):1651-657.

15.FHC Crick, "On protein synthesis", the symposia of the society for experimental Biology.1958;12(1):138-163.

16.F. Crick, "Central Dogma of Molecular Biology," Nature.1970;22(7):561–563.

17.JD Watson and FHC Crick, "Molecular Structure of Nucleic Acids: A Structure for Deoxyribose Nucleic Acid," Nature.1953; 17(1):737–738.

18.J Diamond, "Evolution, consequences and future of plant and animal domestication.," Nature.2002;41(8):700–707.

19.H Temin and S Mitzutani, "Rna-dependent dna polymerase in virions of rous sarcoma virus.," Nature.1970; 22(6):1211–1213.

20.D Baltimore, " RNA-dependent DNA polymerase in virions of RNA tumour viruses.," Nature.1970;22(6):1209–1211.

21.R Gallo, P Sarin, E Gelmann, M Robert-Guroff, E RicharDiabeticon, V Kalyanaraman, D Mann, GSidhu, R Stahl, S Zolla-Pazner, J Leibowitch, and M Popovic, "Isola-tion of human t-cell leukemia virus in acquired immune deficiency syndrome (aids)," Science.1983; 22(4):865–867.

22.F Barre-Sinoussi, J Chermann, F Rey, M Nugeyre, S Chamaret, J Gruest, C Dauguet, C Axler-Blin, F Vezinet-Brun, C Rouzioux, W Rozenbaum, and L Montagnier, "Isolation of a t-lymphotropic retrovirus from a patient at risk for acquired immune deficiency syndrome (aids)," Science. 1983; 22 (9):868–871.

23.C W Greider and E H Blackburn, "Identification of a specific telomere terminal transferase activity in tetrahymena extracts," Cell.1985; 43(2): 405 – 413.

24.D E Gomez, R G Armando, H G Farina, P L Menna, C S Cerrudo, P D Ghiringhelli, and D F Alonso, "Telomere structure and telomerase in health and disease," International Journal ofOncology.2012;41(4):1561–1569.

25.E S Epel, E H Blackburn, J Lin, F S Dhabhar, N E Adler, J D Morrow, and "Accelerated telomere shortening in response to life stress," Proceedings of the National Academy of Sciences of the United States of America.2004;101(49): 17312–17315.

26.M Crous-Bou, T T Fung, J Prescott, B Julin, M Du, Q. Sun, K. M. Rexrode"Mediterranean diet and telomere length in nurses' health study: population based cohort study," BMJ. 2014; 34(9):363-372.

27.D Ornish, J Lin, J M Chan, E Epel, C Kemp, G Weidner, R Marlin, S J Frenda, M J M Magbanus, J Daubenmier, I. Estay, N. K. Hills, N. Chainani-Wu, , "Efect of comprehensive lifestyle changes on telomerase activity and telomere length in men with biopsy-proven low-risk prostate cancer: 5-year follow-up of a descriptive pilot study," The Lancet Oncology. 2013;14 (1): 1112–1120.

28. "Initial sequencing and analysis of the human genome," Nature. 2001; 409 (1):860–921.

29. F Jacobs, D Greenberg, N Nguyen, M Haeussler, A D Ewing, S Katzman, "An evolutionary arms race between KRAB zinc-finger genes ZNF91/93 and SVA/L1 retrotransposons," Nature.2014; 51(6): 242–245.

30. R Cordaux and M. A. Batzer, "The impact of retrotransposons on human genome evolution," Nat Rev Genet.2009; 10 (2):691–703.

31. J. C. Alwine, D. J. Kemp, and G. R. Stark, "Method for detection of specific RNAs in agarose gels by transfer to diazobenzyloxymethyl-paper and hybridization with DNA probes," Proceedings of the National Academy of Sciences.1977; 74 (1):5350–5354.

32. E M Southern, "Detection of specific sequences among DNA fragments separated by gel electrophoresis.," Journal of molecular biology.1975;98 (3):503–517.

33. W F Scherer, J T Syverton, and G Gey, "Studies on the propagation in vitro of poliomyelitis viruses: Iv. viral multiplication in a stable strain of human malignant epithelial cells (strain hela) derived from an epidermoid carcinoma of the cervix," The Journal of Experimental Medicine. 1953; 97 (5): 695–710.

34. R Skloot,L W Hugerth, J Larsson, J Alneberg, M V Lindh, C Legrand, J Pinhassi, and F Andersson, "Metagenome-assembled genomes uncover a global brackish micro-biome," Genome Biology.2015;16(1):1–18.

35. BB Matijašić, T Obermajer, L Lipoglavšek, I Grabnar, G Avguštin, and I Rogelj, "Association of dietary type with fecal microbiota in vegetarians and omnivores in slovenia," European Journal of Nutrition. 2013; 53(4):1051–1064.

36. Levy S, Sutton G, Ng PC, et al. The diploid genome sequence of an individual human. PLoS Biol.2007; 5 (10):245- 254.

37. Feuk L, Carson AR, Scherer SW. Structural variation in the human genome. Nat Rev Genet 2006; 7(1): 85-97.

38. Iafrate AJ, Feuk L, Rivera MN, et al. Detection of large-scale variation in the human genome.Nat Genet.2004; 36 (2): 949-51.\

39. Estivill X, Armengol L. Copy number variants and common disorders: filling the gaps andexploring complexity in genome-wide association studies. PLoS Genet 2007; 3 (1): 1787-99.

40. Doria A, Patti ME, Kahn CR. The emerging genetic architecture of type 2 diabetes. Cell Metab.2008; 8 (1): 186-200.

41. Mangin B, Siberchicot A, Nicolas S, Doligez A, This P, Cierco-Ayrolles C. Novel measures of linkage disequilibrium that correct the bias due to population structure

and relatedness. Heredity.2011; 108 (3):285-91.

42. Pasaniuc B, Avinery R, Gur T, Skibola CF, Bracci PM, Halperin E. A generic coalescent-based framework for the selection of a reference panel for imputation. Genet Epidemiol.2010; 34 (1):773-82.

43. Hattersley AT, McCarthy MI. What makes a good genetic association study? Lancet.2005; 36 (6): 1315-23.

44. Hopper JL, Bishop DT, Easton DF. Population-based family studies in genetic epidemiology. Lancet.2005; 36(6): 1397-406.

45. McCarthy MI. Growing evidence for diabetes susceptibility genes from genome scan data. Curr Diab Rep. 2003; 3(1): 159-67.

46. Vaxillaire M, Froguel P. Genetic basis of maturity-onset diabetes of the young. Endocrinol Metab Clin North Am.2006; 35 (1): 371-84.

47. Waterfield T, Gloyn AL, Monogenic ù-cell dysfunction in children: clinical phenotypes, genetic etiology and mutational pathways. Pediatric Health.2008; 2(4):255-62.

48. O'Rahilly S. Human genetics illuminates the pathealthy to metabolic disease. Nature.2009; 46(2):307-14.

49. Lander ES, Schork NJ. Genetic dissection of complex traits. Science.1994;26(5):2037-48.

50. Risch NJ. Searching for genetic determinants in the new millennium. Nature.2000; 40(5): 847-56.

51. Lohmueller KE, Pearce CL, Pike M, Lander ES, Hirschhorn JN. Meta-analysis of genetic association studies supports a contribution of common variants to susceptibility to common disease. Nat Genet.2003; 33(1): 177-82.

52. Ioannidis JP, Ntzani EE, Trikalinos TA, Contopoulos-Ioannidis DG. Replication validity of genetic association studies. Nat Genet.2001; 2 (9): 306-9.

53. Ioannidis JP. Why most published research findings are false. PLoS Med.2005; 2(1):124-128.

54. Zondervan KT, Cardon LR. The complex interplay among factors that influence allelic association. Nat Rev Genet.2004; 5 (1): 89-100.

55. Risch N, Merikangas K. The future of genetic studies of complex human diseases. Science.1996; 27(3): 1516-27.

56. Reich DE, Lander ES. On the allelic spectrum of human disease. TrenDiabetic Genet.2001; 17(3): 502-10.

57. Petretto E, Liu ET, Aitman TJ. A gene harvest revealing the archeology and complexity of human disease. Nat Genet.2007; 3(9):1299-301.

58. Lander ES, Linton LM, Birren B, et al. Initial sequencing and analysis of the human genome. Nature.2001; 40(9): 860-921.

59. Venter JC, Adams MD, Myers EW, et al. The sequence of the human genome. Science. 2001; 29(1):1304-51.

60. Frazer KA, Ballinger DG, Cox DR, et al. A second generation human haplotype map of over 3.1 million SNPs. Nature.2007; 44(9): 851-61.

61. Hindorff LA, Sethupathy P, Junkins HA, Ramos EM, Mehta JP, Collins FS, Manolio TA. Potential etiologic and functional implications of genome-wide association loci for human diseases and traits. Proc Natl Acad Sci U S A. 200);10(6):9326-37.

62. Lyssenko V, Nagorny CL, Erdos MR, et al. Common variant in MTNR1B associated with increased risk of type 2 diabetes and impaired early insulin secretion. Nat Genet.2009; 4()1: 82-88.

63. Prokopenko I, Langenberg C, Florez JC, et al. Variants in MTNR1B influence fasting glucose levels. Nat Genet.2009; 4(1):77-81.

64. Jacq, C, Miller J and Brownlee G "A pseudogene structure in 5S DNA of Xenopus Laevis". Cell.1977;12(4):109-120.

65. Mighell, A.J, Smith, N.R "Vertebrate Pseudogenes." FEBS Lett.2000; 46(8):109-114.

66. Zhang, Z.D., Frankish A,.Hunt T "Identification and analysis of unitary pseudogenes: historic andcontemporary gene losses in humans and other primates," genome biology.2010; 11(3), 26-34.

67. D.Eisenberg, E.M.MArcotte, I.Xenarios, and T.O.Yeates. Protein function in the post genomic era.Nature.2000; 40(5): 823-36.

68. E.S. Lander, and etal. Initial sequencing and analysis of the human genome. Nature.2001; 40(9):860-921.

69. B.Albert and et al Molecular Biology of the cell. Garland Publishing inc.,New York, NY.1994;3(2) edition.

70. A Pandey and M Mann. Proteomics to study genes and genomes., Nature.2000; 405 (6788) :837-46.

71. A Hamosh, AF Scott, and Et al. online mendelian inheritance in man (OMIM), a knowledgebaseof human genes and genetic disorders. Nucleic Acids.2002; 30 (1): 52-55.

72. A Bairoch and Et al. The SWISS-PROT protein sequence data bank. Nucleic Acids 1991; 19(2): 2247-9.

73. DJ Lockhart and E AWinze;er. Genomics, gene expression and DNA Arrays.

Nature.2000; 405(6788):827-36.

74. D A Benson, DJ Lipman and Et al, Genbank. Nucleic Acids.2002;30 (1): 17-20.

75. G Stoesser, W Baker, and Et al The EMBL nucleotide sequence database. Nucleic Acids2002;30(1): 21-26.

76. Y Tateno, S Miyakazi and Et al, DNA Databank of Japan (DDBJ) for genome scale research in life science. Nucleic Acids.2002; 30 (1): 27-30.

77. M D Adams, J Kelley, and Et al, Complementary DNA Sequencing: expressed sequence tags and human genome project. Science.1991; 252 (5013): 1651-56.

78. M.D. Adams, J.m Kelley, and Et al, Initial assessment of human gene diversity and expression patterns based upon 83 million nucleotides of cDNA Sequence. Nature.1995; 377 (6547):163-174.

79. A Christoffels, and Et al Sequence tag alignment and consensus knowledgebase. Nucleic AcidsRes.2001; 29 (1): 234-38.

80. A Bairoch and RApweiler, The swiss-prot protein sequence database and its supplement TrEMBLin 2000. Nucleic Acids Res. 2000; 28 (1):45-8.

81. X Wen, S Fuhrman and Et al, Large scale temporal gene expression mapping of central nervoussystem development. Proc Natl Acad. Sci USA.1998; 95 (1): 334-9.

82. V E Velculescu, B Vogelstein and Et al, Analysis uncharted transcriptomes with SAGE. Trends Genet. 2000; 16(10): 423-5.

83. M Schena, D Schalon, RW Davis, Quantitative monitoring of gene Expression patterns with a complementary DNA Microarray. Science. 1995;270(5235):467-70.

84. P O Brown and D Botstein. Exploring the new world of the genome with DNA microarrays. Nat Genet.1999; 21 (1): 33-7.

85. B Alberts, A Johnson, J Lewis, K Roberts M Raff, and P Walter. *Molecular Biology of the Cell*. Garland, 2002; 12 (1): 139-152.

86. U Alon, N Barkai, D A Notterman, K Gish, S Ybarra, D Mack, and A J Levine. Broad patterns of gene expression revealed by clustering analysis of tumor and normal colon tissues probed by oligonucleotide arrays. *Proceedings of the National Academy of Science*. 1999;96(12):6745–50.

87. Alter, P Brown, and D Botstein. Singular value decomposition for genome-wide ex-pression data processing and modeling. *Proceedings of the National Academy of Science* 2000; 100(6):3351–6.

88. Z Bar-Joseph, G K Gerber, DK Gifford, TS Jaakkola, and I Simon. Continuous represen-tations of time-series gene expression data. *Journal of Computational Biology*.2003; 10(4):241– 256.

89. Y Barash and N Friedman. Context-speci c Bayesian clustering for gene expression data. *Journal of Computational Biology*. 2002; 9(2):169–191.

90. G Chisholm and TG Cooper. Isolation and characterization of mutants that produce the allantoin- degrading enzymes constitutively in saccharomyces cerevisiae. *Mol Cell Biol*. 1982; 2(9):1088–95.

91. The Gene Ontology Consortium. Gene ontology: tool for the uni cation of biology. *Nature Genetics*.2000; 25(1):25–29.

92. G Cooper and C Yoo. Causal discovery from a mixture of experimental and observational data. In *Proceedings of the Fifteenth Annual Conference on Uncertainty in Arti cial Intelli-gence (UAI)*. 1999; 14(2):116–125.

93. G. F. Cooper and E. Herskovits. A Bayesian method for the induction of probabilistic net-works from data. *Machine Learning*.1992; 9(3):309–347.

94. G F Cooper and C. Glymour. *Computation, Causation, and Discovery*. MIT Press,1999.

95. TH Cormen, CE Leiserson, RL Rivest, and C Stein. *Introduction to Algorithms*. MIT press, 2001.

96. M B Eisen, P T Spellman, P O Brown, and D Botstein. Cluster analysis and display of genome- wide expression patterns. *Proceedings of the National Academy of Science*.1998; 9(5):14863–14868.

97. G Elidan and N Friedman. Learning the dimensionality of hidden variables. In *Proceedings of the Seventeenth Annual Conference on Uncertainty in Arti cial Intelligence (UAI)*.2001; 5 (7): 144–151.

98. G Elidan, N Lotner, N Friedman, and D Koller. Discovering hidden variables: A structure-based approach. In *Proceedings of Neural Information Processing Systems (NIPS)*.2000;3(1):479–485.

99. N Friedman and M Goldsmith. Learning Bayesian networks with local structure. In M. I. Jordan, editor, *Learning in Graphical Models*.1998;421–460.

100. Friedman, I Nachman, and D Pe'er. Learning Bayesian network structure from massive datasets:The "sparse candidate" algorithm. In *Proceedings of the Fifteenth Annual Confer-ence on Uncertainty inArtificial Intelligence (UAI)*.1999;196–205.

101. N Friedman and Z Yakhini. On the sample complexity of learning Bayesian networks. In *Proceedings of the Twelfth Annual Conference on Uncertainty in Arti cial Intelligence (UAI)*.1996; 274–282.

102. A P Gasch, P T Spellman, C M Kao, O Carmel-Harel, M B Eisen, G Storz, D Botstein, and P O Brown. Genomic expression program in the response of yeast cells to environmental changes. *Mol. Bio. Cell*.2000;11 (5):4241–4257.

103. D. Geiger and D. Heckerman. Learning gaussian networks. *In Proceedings of the Tenth AnnualConference on Uncertainty in Artifi cial Intelligence* (UAI) 1994; 2 (1): 235–243.

104. A J Hartemink, DK Gifford, TS Jaakkola, and RA Young. Combining location and ex-pression data for principled discovery of genetic regulatory networks. In *Paci c Symposium on Biocomputing*.2002; 4 (3): 437–449.

105. D Heckerman and D Geiger. Learning Bayesian networks: a uni cation for discrete and Gaussian domains. In *Proceedings of the Eleventh Annual Conference on Uncertainty in Arti cial Intelligence (UAI)*.1995; 5 (2): 274–284.

106. D Heckerman, D Geiger, and D Chickering. Learning Bayesian networks: The combi-nation of knowledge and statistical data. In *Proceedings of the Tenth Annual Conference on Uncertainty in Arti cial Intelligence (UAI)*.1994; 6 (3): 293–301.

107. D. Heckerman, C. Meek, and G. Cooper. A Bayesian approach to causal discovery. In *Computation, Causation, and Discovery*.1996;19 (2):141–166.

108. NS. Holter, M Mitra, A Maritan, M Cieplak, JR. Banavar, and NV. Fedoroff. Fundamental patterns underlying gene expression pro le: Simplicity from complexity. *Proceedings of the National Academy of Science*.2000; 97 (8): 8409–14.

109. T Hughes, M Marton, A Jones, C Roberts, R Stoughton, C Armour, H Bennett, E Coffey, H Dai, Y He, M Kidd, A King, M Meyer, D Slade, P Lum, S Stepaniants, D Shoemaker, D Gachotte, K Chakraburtty, J Simon, M Bard, and S Friend. Functional discovery via a compendium of expression pro les. *Cell*.2000; 102(1):109–26.

110. T Ideker, O Ozier, B Schwikowski, and A Siegel. Discovering regulatory and signal-ing circuits in molecular interaction networks. In *ProceedinDiabetic of the Tenth International Conference onIntelligent Systems for Molecular Biology.* 2002; 5(3):233–240.

111. V Iyer, M Eisen, D Ross, G Schuler, T Moore, J Lee, J Trent, M Staudt, JR, The trasncriptional program in the response of human broblasts to serum. Science.1999; 283 (5398): 83-7.

112. J Jaffe, H Berg, and G Church. Proteogenomic mapping reveals genomic structure and novel proteins undetected by computational algorithms. *Proteomics*, 2003.

113. F V Jensen. *An introduction to Bayesian Networks*. University College London Press, London.1996.

114. M Kellis, N Patterson, M Endrizzi, B Birren, and E Lander. Sequencing and

comparison of yeast species to identify genes and regulatory elements. *Nature*. 2003; 4(23):241–54.

115. Liu M,. Hu BL, Cui LY. "Clinical and neurophysiological features of 700 patients with diabetic peripheral neuropathy." Zhonghua Nei Ke Za Zhi. 2005; 4(4): 173-6.

116. Chadha V, Shivalkar SS, "Does Body Mass Index Effect Nerve Conduction ? A cross sectional study" IJCRR. 2016;8(7): 04-7.

117. Callaghan BC, Xia R, ReynolDiabetic E, "Association Between Metabolic Syndrome Components and polyneuropathy in an obese population." JAMA Neurol. 2016; 4 (5): 1231-239.

118. Permutt MA, Wasson J, Cox N. Genetic epidemiology of diabetes. J Clin Invest.2005; 1(15): 1431-9.

119. Diagnosis and classification of diabetes mellitus. Diabetes Care.2011; 34(1): 62-9.

120. Alberti KG, Zimmet PZ. Definition, diagnosis and classification of diabetes mellitus and its complications. Part 1: diagnosis and classification of diabetes mellitus provisional report of a WHO consultation. Diabet Med 1998; 1(5): 539-53.

121. Shaw JE, Sicree RA, Zimmet PZ. Global estimates of the prevalence of diabetes for 2010 and 2030. Diabetes Res Clin Pract.2009; 8(7): 4-14.

122. Midthjell K, Kruger O, Holmen J, Tverdal A, Claudi T, Bjorndal A, Magnus P. Rapid changes in the prevalence of obesity and known diabetes in an adult Norwegian population. The Nord-Trondelag Health Surveys: 1984-1986 and 1995-1997. Diabetes Care 1999; 2(2): 1813-20.

123. Stene LC, Midthjell K, Jenum AK, et al. [Prevalence of diabetes mellitus in Norway]. TiDiabeticskr Nor Laegeforen. 2004; 12(4): 1511-4.

124. Report of the Expert Committee on the Diagnosis and Classification of Diabetes Mellitus. Diabetes Care 1997; 20: 1183-97.

125. Report of the expert committee on the diagnosis and classification of diabetes mellitus. Diabetes Care 2003; 26 (1): 5-20.

126. WHO/International Diabetes Federation. Definition and diagnosis of diabetes mellitus and intermediate hyperglycemia: report of a WHO/IDF consultation.2006.

127. Intensive blood-glucose control with sulphonylureas or insulin compared with conventional treatment and risk of complications in patients with type 2 diabetes (UKPREDIABETIC 33). UK Prospective Diabetes Study (UKPREDIABETIC) Group. Lancet.1998; 35(2): 837-53.

128. Khaw KT, Wareham N. Glycated hemoglobin as a marker of cardiovascular risk.

Curr Opin Lipidol 2006; 17: 637-43.

129. Pradhan AD, Rifai N, Buring JE, Ridker PM. Hemoglobin A1c predicts diabetes but not cardiovascular disease in nondiabetic women. Am J Med 2007; 120: 720-7.

130. Murphy R, Ellard S, Hattersley AT. Clinical implications of a molecular genetic classification of monogenic beta-cell diabetes. Nat Clin Pract Endocrinol Metab 2008; 4: 200-13.

131. Online Mendelian Inheritance in Man, OMIM. Baltimore, MD. MIM Number: 606391: Accessed Johns Hopkins University.2011; 9 (2):11-23.

132. Eide SA, Raeder H, Johansson S, Midthjell K, Sovik O, Njolstad PR, Molven A. Prevalence of HNF1A (MODY3) mutations in a Norwegian population (the HUNT2 Study). Diabet Med. 2008; 25: 775-81.

133. Njolstad PR, Hertel JK, Sovik O, Raeder H, Johansson S, Molven A. [Progress in diabetesgenetics]. TiDiabeticskr Nor Laegeforen 2010; 130: 1145-9.

134. De Leon DD, Stanley CA. Permanent Neonatal Diabetes Mellitus. In: Pagon RA, ed, GeneReviews. Seattle (WA): University of Washington, Seattle.1993: 5 (8), 2422-436.

135. Njolstad PR, Sagen JV, Bjorkhaug L, et al. Permanent neonatal diabetes caused by glucokinase deficiency: inborn error of the glucose-insulin signaling pathway. Diabetes 2003; 52: 2854-60.

136. Pearson ER, Flechtner I, Njolstad PR, et al. Switching from insulin to oral sulfonylureas in patientswith diabetes due to Kir6.2 mutations. N Engl J Med 2006; 355: 467-77.

137. Sagen JV, Raeder H, Hathout E, et al. Permanent neonatal diabetes due to mutations in KCNJ11 encoding Kir6.2: patient characteristics and initial response to sulfonylurea therapy. Diabetes 2004; 53: 2713-8.

138. Jones CW. Gestational diabetes and its impact on the neonate. Neonatal Netw 2001; 20: 17-23.

139. Metzger BE, Lowe LP, Dyer AR, et al. Hyperglycemia and adverse pregnancy outcomes. N Engl JMed 2008; 358: 991-02.

140. Lobner K, Knopff A, Baumgarten A, et al. Predictors of postpartum diabetes in women with gestational diabetes mellitus. Diabetes 2006; 55: 792-7.

141. Boney CM, Verma A, Tucker R, Vohr BR. Metabolic syndrome in childhood: association with birth weight, maternal obesity, and gestational diabetes mellitus. Pediatrics 2005; 115: 290-6.

142. Eckel RH, Kahn SE, Ferrannini E, et al. Obesity and type 2 diabetes: what can be unified and whatneeds to be individualized? Diabetes Care.2011; 34:1242-30.

143. Wang J, Luben R, Khaw KT, Bingham S, Wareham NJ, Forouhi NG. Dietary energy density predicts the risk of incident type 2 diabetes: the European Prospective Investigation of Cancer (EPIC)- Norfolk Study. Diabetes Care.2008; 31: 2120-5.

144. Hectors TL, Vanparys C, van der Ven K, et al. Environmental pollutants and type 2 diabetes: a review of mechanisms that can disrupt beta cell function. Diabetologia 2011; 54: 1273-90.

145. Anderson JW, Kendall CW, Jenkins DJ. Importance of weight management in type 2 diabetes: review with meta-analysis of clinical studies. J Am Coll Nutr 2003; 22: 331-9.

146. Schulze MB, Heidemann C, Schienkiewitz A, Bergmann MM, Hoffmann K, Boeing H. Comparison of anthropometric characteristics in predicting the incidence of type 2 diabetes in the EPIC- Potsdam study. Diabetes Care 2006; 29: 1921-3.

147. Pierce M, Keen H, Bradley C. Risk of diabetes in offspring of parents with non-insulin-dependent diabetes. Diabet Med 1995; 12: 6-13.

148. Shai I, Jiang R, Manson JE, Stampfer MJ, Willett WC, Colditz GA, Hu FB. Ethnicity, obesity, andrisk of type 2 diabetes in women: a 20-year follow-up study. Diabetes Care 2006; 29: 1585-90.

149. Nichols GA, Hillier TA, Brown JB. Progression from newly acquired impaired fasting glusose to type 2 diabetes. Diabetes Care 2007; 30: 228-33.

150. Gress TW, Nieto FJ, Shahar E, Wofford MR, Brancati FL. Hypertension and antihypertensive therapy as risk factors for type 2 diabetes mellitus. Atherosclerosis Risk in Communities Study. N Engl JMed 2000; 342: 905-12.

151. Mooradian AD. Dyslipidemia in type 2 diabetes mellitus. Nat Clin Pract Endocrinol Metab 2009; 5: 150-9.

152. Hu FB, Manson JE, Stampfer MJ, Colditz G, Liu S, Solomon CG, Willett WC. Diet, lifestyle, and the risk of type 2 diabetes mellitus in women. N Engl J Med. 2001; 345: 790-7.

153. Kim C, Newton KM, Knopp RH. Gestational diabetes and the incidence of type 2 diabetes: a systematic review. Diabetes Care 2002; 25: 1862-8.

154. Whincup PH, Kaye SJ, Owen CG, et al. Birth weight and risk of type 2 diabetes: a systematic review. JAMA. 2008; 300: 2886-97.

155. Legro RS. Type 2 diabetes and polycystic ovary syndrome. Fertil Steril 2006; 86(1): S16-7.

156. DECODE Study Group: Age- and sex-specific prevalences of diabetes and impaired glucose regulation in 13 European cohorts. Diabetes Care.2003; 26: 61-9.

157. Dechenes CJ, Verchere CB, Andrikopoulos S, Kahn SE. Human aging is associated with parallel reductions in insulin and amylin release. Am J Physiol 1998; 275: E785-91.

158. Bloomgarden ZT. Type 2 diabetes in the young: the evolving epidemic. Diabetes Care 2004; 27: 998-1010.

159. International Diabetes Federation. IDF Diabetes Atlas, 4th edn. Brussels, Belgium: International Diabetes Federation.2009.

160. Boden G. Fatty acids and insulin resistance. Diabetes Care.1996; 19: 394-5.

161. Rabe K, Lehrke M, Parhofer KG, Broedl UC. Adipokines and insulin resistance. Mol Med 2008; 14: 741-51.

162. Kim JA, Wei Y, Sowers JR. Role of mitochondrial dysfunction in insulin resistance. Circ Res 2008; 102: 401-14.

163. Robertson RP, Harmon J, Tran PO, Tanaka Y, Takahashi H. Glucose toxicity in beta-cells: type 2 diabetes, good radicals gone bad, and the glutathione connection. Diabetes.2003; 52: 581-7.

164. Robertson RP, Harmon J, Tran PO, Poitout V. Beta-cell glucose toxicity, lipotoxicity, and chronic oxidative stress in type 2 diabetes. Diabetes 2004; 53 (1): S119-24.

165. Hull RL, Westermark GT, Westermark P, Kahn SE. Islet amyloid: a critical entity in the pathogenesis of type 2 diabetes. J Clin Endocrinol Metab 2004; 89:3629-43.

166. Stumvoll M, GolDiabetictein BJ, van Haeften TW. Type 2 diabetes: principles of pathogenesis and therapy. Lancet.2005; 365: 1333-46.

167. Haffner SM, D'Agostino R, Jr., Mykkanen L, et al. Insulin sensitivity in subjects with type 2 diabetes. Relationship to cardiovascular risk factors: the Insulin Resistance Atherosclerosis Study. Diabetes Care.1999; 22: 562-8.

168. Stern MP. Do non-insulin-dependent diabetes mellitus and cardiovascular disease share common antecedents? Ann Intern Med.1996; 124: 110-6.

169. Nathan DM, Buse JB, DaviDiabeticon MB, Ferrannini E, Holman RR, Sherwin R, Zinman B. Medical management of hyperglycemia in type 2 diabetes: a consensus algorithm for the initiation and adjustment of therapy: a consensus statement of the American Diabetes Association and the European Association for the Study of Diabetes. Diabetes Care.2009; 32: 193-203.

170. Nathan DM, Cleary PA, Backlund JY, et al. Intensive diabetes treatment and cardiovascular disease in patients with type 1 diabetes. N Engl J Med.2005; 1 (5): 2643-53.

171. Taubes G. Diabetes. Paradoxical effects of tightly controlled blood sugar. Science

2008; 322: 365- 7.

172. Monti MC, Lonsdale JT, Montomoli C, Montross R, Schlag E, Greenberg DA. Familial risk factors for microvascular complications and differential male-female risk in a large cohort of American families with type 1 diabetes. J Clin Endocrinol Metab 2007; 92: 4650-5.

173. Reaven G. The metabolic syndrome or the insulin resistance syndrome? Different names, different concepts, and different goals. Endocrinol Metab Clin North Am.2004; 33: 283-303.

174. Zimmet P, Alberti KG, Shaw J. Global and societal implications of the diabetes epidemic. Nature.2001; 414: 782-7.

175. Altshuler D, Daly MJ, Lander ES. Genetic mapping in human disease. Science.2008; 322: 881-8.

176. Groop L, Lyssenko V, "Genetics of Type 2 Diabetes. An Overview." Endocrinol. Nutrition. 2009;56(09): 73515-526.

177. Poulsen P, Kyvik KO, Vaag A, Beck-Nielsen H. Heritability of type II (non-insulin-dependent) diabetes mellitus and abnormal glucose tolerance--a population-based twin study. Diabetologia 1999;42: 139-45.

178. Mangin B, Siberchicot A, Nicolas S, Doligez A, This P, Cierco-Ayrolles C. Novel measures of linkage disequilibrium that correct the bias due to population structure and relatedness. Heredity 2011; 7(2): 235-240 .

179. Almgren P, Lehtovirta M, Isomaa B, et al. Heritability and familiality of type 2 diabetes and related quantitative traits in the Botnia Study. Diabetologia 2011; 3(1): 785-95.

180. Lillioja S, Wilton A. Agreement among type 2 diabetes linkage studies but a poor correlation with results from genome-wide association studies. Diabetologia.2009; 5(2): 1061-74.

181. Grant SF, Thorleifsson G, Reynisdottir I, et al. Variant of transcription factor 7-like2 (TCF7L2) gene confers risk of type 2 diabetes. Nat Genet.2006; 3(8):320-3.

182. Frayling TM. Genome-wide association studies provide new insights into type 2 diabetes aetiology. Nat Rev Genet.2007; 8: 657-62.

183. Florez JC, Burtt N, de Bakker PI, et al. Haplotype structure and genotype-phenotype correlations of the sulfonylurea receptor and the islet ATP-sensitive potassium channel gene region. Diabetes.2004; 5(3): 1360-8.

184. Nielsen EM, Hansen L, Carstensen B, et al. The E23K variant of Kir6.2 associates with impaired post-OGTT serum insulin response and increased risk of type 2 diabetes. Diabetes.2003; 5(2): 573-7.

185. Altshuler D, Hirschhorn JN, Klannemark M, et al. The common PPARgamma Pro12Ala polymorphism is associated with decreased risk of type 2 diabetes. Nat Genet (2000); 26: 76-80.

186. Sandhu MS, Weedon MN, Fawcett KA, et al. Common variants in WFS1 confer risk of type 2 diabetes. Nat Genet.2007;402: 880-93.

187. GudmunDiabeticson J, Sulem P, Steinthorsdottir V, et al. Two variants on chromosome 17 confer prostate cancer risk, and the one in TCF2 protects against type 2 diabetes. Nat Genet 2007; 39: 977-83.

188. Winckler W, Weedon MN, Graham RR, et al. Evaluation of common variants in the six known maturity-onset diabetes of the young (MODY) genes for association with type 2 diabetes. Diabetes.2007;56: 685-93.

189. Barroso I, Gurnell M, Crowley VE, et al. Dominant negative mutations in human PPARgamma associated with severe insulin resistance, diabetes mellitus and hypertension. Nature 1999; 402: 880-3.

190. Gloyn AL, Pearson ER, Antcliff JF, et al. Activating mutations in the gene encoding the ATP- sensitive potassium-channel subunit Kir6.2 and permanent neonatal diabetes. N Engl J Med.2004; 350: 1838-49.

191. Inoue H, Tanizawa Y, Wasson J, et al. A gene encoding a transmembrane protein is mutated in patients with diabetes mellitus and optic atrophy (Wolfram syndrome). Nat Genet 1998; 20: 143-8.

192. Nishigori H, Yamada S, Kohama T, et al. Frameshift mutation, A263fsinsGG, in the hepatocyte nuclear factor-1beta gene associated with diabetes and renal dysfunction. Diabetes.1998; 47: 1354-5.

193. Saxena R, Voight BF, Lyssenko V, et al. Genome-wide association analysis identifies loci for type2 diabetes and triglyceride levels. Science.2007; 316: 1331-6.

194. Scott LJ, Mohlke KL, Bonnycastle LL, et al. A genome-wide association study of type 2 diabetes in Finns detects multiple susceptibility variants. Science 2007; 316: 1341-5.

195. Sladek R, Rocheleau G, Rung J, et al. A genome-wide association study identifies novel risk loci for type 2 diabetes. Nature.2007; 445: 881-5.

196. Steinthorsdottir V, Thorleifsson G, Reynisdottir I, et al. A variant in CDKAL1 influences insulin response and risk of type 2 diabetes. Nat Genet.2007; 39: 770-5.

197. Zeggini E, Weedon MN, Lindgren CM, et al. Replication of genome-wide association signals in UK samples reveals risk loci for type 2 diabetes. Science.2007; 316: 1336-41.

198. Florez JC, Manning AK, Dupuis J, et al. A 100K genome-wide association scan for diabetes and related traits in the Framingham Heart Study: replication and integration with other genome-widedatasets. Diabetes.2007; 56: 3063-74.

199. Hanson RL, Bogardus C, Duggan D, et al. A search for variants associated with young-onset type 2 diabetes in American Indians in a 100K genotyping array. Diabetes 2007; 56: 3045-52.

200. Hayes MG, Pluzhnikov A, Miyake K, et al. Identification of type 2 diabetes genes in Mexican Americans through genome-wide association studies. Diabetes.2007; 56: 3033-44.

201. Rampersaud E, Damcott CM, Fu M, et al. Identification of novel candidate genes for type 2 diabetes from a genome-wide association scan in the Old Order Amish: evidence for replication from diabetes-related quantitative traits and from independent populations. Diabetes 2007; 56: 3053-62.

202. Salonen JT, Uimari P, Aalto JM, et al. Type 2 diabetes whole-genome association study in four populations: the DiaGen consortium. Am J Hum Genet.2007; 81: 338-45.

203. Cauchi S, Meyre D, Dina C, et al. Transcription factor TCF7L2 genetic study in the French population: expression in human beta-cells and adipose tissue and strong association with type 2 diabetes. Diabetes.2006; 55: 2903-8.

204. Chandak GR, Janipalli CS, Bhaskar S, et al. Common variants in the TCF7L2 gene are strongly associated with type 2 diabetes mellitus in the Indian population. Diabetologia.2007; 50: 63-7.

205. Damcott CM, Pollin TI, Reinhart LJ, et al. Polymorphisms in the transcription factor 7-like 2 (TCF7L2) gene are associated with type 2 diabetes in the Amish: replication and evidence for a role in both insulin secretion and insulin resistance. Diabetes.2006; 55: 2654-9.

206. Florez JC, Jablonski KA, Bayley N, et al. TCF7L2 polymorphisms and progression to diabetes in the Diabetes Prevention Program. N Engl J Med.2006; 355: 241-50.

207. Groves CJ, Zeggini E, Minton J, et al. Association analysis of 6,736 U.K. subjects provides replication and confirms TCF7L2 as a type 2 diabetes susceptibility gene with a substantial effect on individual risk. Diabetes.2006; 55: 2640-4.

208. Hayashi T, Iwamoto Y, Kaku K, Hirose H, Maeda S. Replication study for the association of TCF7L2 with susceptibility to type 2 diabetes in a Japanese population. Diabetologia.2007; 50: 980-4.

209. Humphries SE, Gable D, Cooper JA, et al. Common variants in the TCF7L2 gene

and predisposition to type 2 diabetes in UK European Whites, Indian Asians and Afro-Caribbean men and women. J Mol Med. 2006; 84: 1-10.

210. Lehman DM, Hunt KJ, Leach RJ, et al. Haplotypes of transcription factor 7-like 2 (TCF7L2) gene and its upstream region are associated with type 2 diabetes and age of onset in Mexican Americans. Diabetes.2007; 56: 389-93.

211. Saxena R, Gianniny L, Burtt NP, et al. Common single nucleotide polymorphisms in TCF7L2 are reproducibly associated with type 2 diabetes and reduce the insulin response to glucose in nondiabetic individuals. Diabetes.2006; 55: 2890-5.

212. Zhang C, Qi L, Hunter DJ, Meigs JB, Manson JE, van Dam RM, Hu FB. Variant of transcription factor 7-like 2 (TCF7L2) gene and the risk of type 2 diabetes in large cohorts of U.S. women and men. Diabetes.2006; 55: 2645-8.

213. Lyssenko V, Lupi R, Marchetti P, et al. Mechanisms by which common variants in the TCF7L2 gene increase risk of type 2 diabetes. J Clin Invest. 2007; 117: 2155-63.

214. The Wellcome Trust Case Control ConsortiumGenome-wide association study of 14,000 cases of seven common diseases and 3,000 shared controls. Nature.2007; 447: 661-78.

215. Helgadottir A, Thorleifsson G, Manolescu A, et al. A common variant on chromosome 9p21 affects the risk of myocardial infarction. Science.2007; 316: 1491-3.

216. McPherson R, Pertsemlidis A, Kavaslar N, et al. A common allele on chromosome 9 associated with coronary heart disease. Science.2007; 316: 1488-91.

217. Samani NJ, Erdmann J, Hall AS, et al. Genomewide association analysis of coronary artery disease. N Engl J Med 2007; 357: 443-53.

218. Helgadottir A, Thorleifsson G, Magnusson KP, et al. The same sequence variant on 9p21 associates with myocardial infarction, abdominal aortic aneurysm and intracranial aneurysm. Nat Genet.2008; 40: 217-24.

219. Matarin M, Brown WM, Singleton A, Hardy JA, Meschia JF. Whole genome analyses suggest ischemic stroke and heart disease share an association with polymorphisms on chromosome 9p21. Stroke. 2008; 39: 1586-9.

220. Newton-Cheh C, Cook NR, VanDenburgh M, Rimm EB, Ridker PM, Albert CM. A common variant at 9p21 is associated with sudden and arrhythmic cardiac death. Circulation.2009; 120: 2062-8.

221. Duesing K, Fatemifar G, Charpentier G, et al. Strong association of common

variants in the CDKN2A/CDKN2B region with type 2 diabetes in French EuropiDiabetic. Diabetologia.2008; 51: 821- 6.

222. Horikawa Y, Miyake K, Yasuda K, et al. Replication of genome-wide association studies of type 2diabetes susceptibility in Japan. J Clin Endocrinol Metab 2008; 93: 3136-41.

223. Ng MC, Park KS, Oh B, et al. Implication of genetic variants near TCF7L2, SLC30A8, HHEX, CDKAL1, CDKN2A/B, IGF2BP2, and FTO in type 2 diabetes and obesity in 6,719 Asians. Diabetes. 2008; 57: 2226-33.

224. Wu Y, Li H, Loos RJ, et al. Common variants in CDKAL1, CDKN2A/B, IGF2BP2, SLC30A8,and HHEX/IDE genes are associated with type 2 diabetes and impaired fasting glucose in a Chinese Hanpopulation. Diabetes.2008; 57:2834-42.

225. Assimes TL, Knowles JW, Basu A, et al. Susceptibility locus for clinical and subclinical coronary artery disease at chromosome 9p21 in the multi-ethnic ADVANCE study. Hum Mol Genet. 2008; 17: 2320-8.

226. Hiura Y, Fukushima Y, Yuno M, et al. Validation of the association of genetic variants on chromosome 9p21 and 1q41 with myocardial infarction in a Japanese population. Circ J.2008; 72: 1213- 7.

227. Larson MG, Atwood LD, Benjamin EJ, et al. Framingham Heart Study 100K project: genome- wide associations for cardiovascular disease outcomes. BMC Med Genet.2007; 8(1): S5.

228. Schunkert H, Gotz A, Braund P, et al. Repeated replication and a prospective meta-analysis of the association between chromosome 9p21.3 and coronary artery disease. Circulation 2008; 11(7): 1675-84.

229. Shen GQ, Li L, Rao S, et al. Four SNPs on chromosome 9p21 in a South Korean population implicate a genetic locus that confers high cross-race risk for development of coronary artery disease. Arterioscler Thromb Vasc Biol.2008; 28: 360-5.

230. Shen GQ, Rao S, Martinelli N, et al. Association between four SNPs on chromosome 9p21 and myocardial infarction is replicated in an Italian population. J Hum Genet.2008; 53: 144-50.

231. Zhou L, Zhang X, He M, Cheng L, Chen Y, Hu FB, Wu T. Associations between single nucleotidepolymorphisms on chromosome 9p21 and risk of coronary heart disease in Chinese Han population. Arterioscler Thromb Vasc Biol.2008; 28: 2085-9.

232. Abdullah KG, Li L, Shen GQ, et al. Four SNPS on chromosome 9p21 confer risk to premature, familial CAD and MI in an American Caucasian population

(GeneQuest). Ann Hum Genet.2008; 72: 654-7.

233. Chen Z, Qian Q, Ma G, et al. A common variant on chromosome 9p21 affects the risk of early- onset coronary artery disease. Mol Biol Rep.2009; 36: 889-93.

234. Wahlstrand B, Orho-Melander M, Delling L, et al. The myocardial infarction associated CDKN2A/CDKN2B locus on chromosome 9p21 is associated with stroke independently of coronary events in patients with hypertension. J Hypertens.2009; 27: 769-73.

235. Ye S, Willeit J, Kronenberg F, Xu Q, Kiechl S. Association of genetic variation on chromosome 9p21 with susceptibility and progression of atherosclerosis: a population-based, prospective study. J Am Coll Cardiol.2008; 52: 378-84.

236. Zee RY, Ridker PM. Two common gene variants on chromosome 9 and risk of atherothrombosis. Stroke.2007; 38: e11-22.

237. Doria A, Wojcik J, Xu R, et al. Interaction between poor glycemic control and 9p21 locus on risk of coronary artery disease in type 2 diabetes. JAMA.2008; 300:2389-97.

238. Broadbent HM, Peden JF, Lorkowski S, et al. Susceptibility to coronary artery disease anddiabetes is encoded by distinct, tightly linked SNPs in the ANRIL locus on chromosome 9p. Hum Mol Genet.2008; 17: 806-14.

239. Cunnington MS, Santibanez Koref M, Mayosi BM, Burn J, Keavney B. Chromosome 9p21 SNPs Associated with Multiple Disease Phenotypes Correlate with ANRIL Expression. PLoS Genet.2010; 6: e1000899.

240. Liu Y, Sanoff HK, Cho H, et al. INK4/ARF transcript expression is associated with chromosome 9p21 variants linked to atherosclerosis. PLoS One.2009; 4: e5027.

241. Harismendy O, Notani D, Song X, et al. 9p21 DNA variants associated with coronary artery disease impair interferon-gamma signalling response. Nature.2011; 470: 264-8.

242. Zeggini E, Scott LJ, Saxena R, et al. Meta-analysis of genome-wide association data and large-scale replication identifies additional susceptibility loci for type 2 diabetes. Nat Genet.2008; 40: 638-45.

243. Unoki H, Takahashi A, Kawaguchi T, et al. SNPs in KCNQ1 are associated with susceptibility to type 2 diabetes in East Asian and European populations. Nat Genet.2008; 40: 1098-102.

244. Yasuda K, Miyake K, Horikawa Y, et al. Variants in KCNQ1 are associated with susceptibility to type 2 diabetes mellitus. Nat Genet.2008;40:1092-7.

245. Tsai FJ, Yang CF, Chen CC, et al. A genome-wide association study

identifies susceptibility variants for type 2 diabetes in Han Chinese. PLoS Genet.2010;6:1000847.

246. Florez JC. Newly identified loci highlight beta cell dysfunction as a key cause of type 2 diabetes: where are the insulin resistance genes? Diabetologia.2008;51:1100-10.

247. Rung J, Cauchi S, Albrechtsen A, et al. Genetic variant near IRS1 is associated with type 2 diabetes, insulin resistance and hyperinsulinemia. Nat Genet.2009;41:1110-5.

248. Mulder H, Nagorny CL, Lyssenko V, Groop L. Melatonin receptors in pancreatic islets: goodmorning to a novel type 2 diabetes gene. Diabetologia.2009; 52: 1240-9.

249. Bouatia-Naji N, Bonnefond A, Cavalcanti-Proenca C, et al. A variant near MTNR1B is associated with increased fasting plasma glucose levels and type 2 diabetes risk. Nat Genet.2009; 41: 89-94.

250. Lyssenko V, Nagorny CL, Erdos MR, et al. Common variant in MTNR1B associated with increased risk of type 2 diabetes and impaired early insulin secretion. Nat Genet.2009; 41: 82-8.

251. Prokopenko I, Langenberg C, Florez JC, et al. Variants in MTNR1B influence fasting glucoselevels. Nat Genet.2009; 41: 77-81.

252. Dupuis J, Langenberg C, Prokopenko I, et al. New genetic loci implicated in fasting glucose homeostasis and their impact on type 2 diabetes risk. Nat Genet.2010; 42: 105-16.

253. Kooner JS, Saleheen D, Sim X, et al. Genome-wide association study in individuals of South Asian ancestry identifies six new type 2 diabetes susceptibility loci. Nat Genet.2011; 43: 984-9.

254. Qi L, Cornelis MC, Kraft P, et al. Genetic variants at 2q24 are associated with susceptibility totype 2 diabetes. Hum Mol Genet.2010; 19: 2706-15.

255. Voight BF, Scott LJ, Steinthorsdottir V, et al. Twelve type 2 diabetes susceptibility loci identified through large-scale association analysis. Nat Genet.2010; 42: 579-89.

256. Civelek M, Lusis AJ. Conducting the metabolic syndrome orchestra. Nat Genet.2011; 43: 506-8.

257. Billings LK, Florez JC. The genetics of type 2 diabetes: what have we learned from GWAS? Ann N Y Acad Sci.2010; 1212: 59-77.

258. Lyssenko V, Jonsson A, Almgren P, et al. Clinical risk factors, DNA variants, and the development of type 2 diabetes. N Engl J Med.2008; 359: 2220-32.

259. Hardy J, Singleton A. Genomewide association studies and human disease. N Engl J Med (2009); 360: 1759-68.

260. Hirschhorn JN. Genomewide association studies--illuminating biologic pathways. N Engl J Med.2009; 360: 1699-701.

261. Kraft P, Hunter DJ. Genetic risk prediction--are we there yet? N Engl J Med.2009; 360: 1701-3.

262. Simonis-Bik AM, Nijpels G, van Haeften TW, et al. Gene variants in the novel type 2 diabetes loci CDC123/CAMK1D, THADA, ADAMTS9, BCL11A, and MTNR1B affect different aspects of pancreatic beta-cell function. Diabetes.2009; 59: 293-301.

263. Boesgaard TW, Gjesing AP, Grarup N, et al. Variant near ADAMTS9 known to associate withtype 2 diabetes is related to insulin resistance in offspring of type 2 diabetes patients--EUGENE2 study. PLoS One.2009; 4 (1): e7236.

264. Grarup N, Rose CS, Andersson EA, et al. Studies of association of variants near the HHEX, CDKN2A/B, and IGF2BP2 genes with type 2 diabetes and impaired insulin release in 10,705 Danish subjects: validation and extension of genome-wide association studies. Diabetes.2007; 56: 3105-11.

265. Deeb SS, Fajas L, Nemoto M, et al. A Pro12Ala substitution in PPARgamma2 associated with decreased receptor activity, lower body mass index and improved insulin sensitivity. Nat Genet.1998; 20: 284-7.

266. Yamagata K, Furuta H, Oda N, et al. Mutations in the hepatocyte nuclear factor-4alpha gene in maturity-onset diabetes of the young (MODY1). Nature.1996; 384: 458-60.

267. Barroso I, Luan J, Wheeler E, et al. Population-specific risk of type 2 diabetes conferred by HNF4A P2 promoter variants: a lesson for replication studies. Diabetes.2008; 57: 3161-5.

268. Meigs JB, Manning AK, Fox CS, Florez JC, Liu C, Cupples LA, Dupuis J. Genome-wide association with diabetes-related traits in the Framingham Heart Study. BMC Med Genet.2007; 8 Suppl 1: S16.

269. Paterson AD, Waggott D, Boright AP, et al. A genome-wide association study identifies a novel major locus for glycemic control in type 1 diabetes, as measured by both A1C and glucose. Diabetes.2010; 59: 539-49.

270. Sladek R, Rochelau G, Rung J,, "A genome wide association study identifies novel risk loci for type 2 diabetes."Nature.2007;445:881-885.

271. Scott L. Mohlke K, Bonnycastle L, "A genome wide association study of type 2 diabetes in Finns detect multiple susceptibility variants" science.2007;31(6):1341-

1345.

272. Morris A.P, Voight B.F, Teslovich. T.M, "Large Scale Association analysis provides insight into the genetic architecture and pathophysiology of type 2 Diabetes." Nat Genet.2012;44:981-990.

273. N. McDonough, Palemar Nd, "Genome wide study for diabetes nephropathy genes in African- American." Kidney int.2011; 79: 563-572.

274. Chandrakumar Sathishkumar et al "Linking a role of lncRNAs (long non-coding RNAs) with insulin resistance, accelerated senescence and inflammation in patients with type 2 diabetes". Human Genomics; (2018), 12 (4):01-09.

275. Oliver Kluth, Daniel Matzke, Gunnar Schulze etal "Differential Transcriptome Anlaysis of Diabetes –Resistant and Sensitive mouse Islets reveals significant overlap with human Diabetes susceptibility Genes." Diabetes; December.2014; 6(3):4230-4238.

276. Chandra shekhar Vasamsetty, etal "Gene Expression Analysis of Type 2 Diabetes Mellitus- A study on diabetes with and without parental history"Journal of theoretical and applied Information Technology.2011;27(1):43-53.

277. Stancakova A, Kuulasmaa T, Paananen J, et al.; Association of 18 confirmed susceptibility locifor type 2 diabetes with indices of insulin release, proinsulin conversion, and insulin sensitivity in 5,327 nondiabetic Finnish men. Diabetes.2009;5(8):2129-36.

278. Jong Wook Choi, Shinje Moon, "Association of prediabetes associated single nucleotide polymorphisms with microalbuminuria" PloS ONE.2017;12(2): e0171367.

279. Andrey E Brown, Mark Walker "Genetics of insulin resistance and the metabolic syndrome"Current Cardiol Rep.2016;1(8):451-464.

280. Rashmi B Prasad, Leif Groop, "Genetics of Type 2 Diabetes-pitfalls and possibilities." Genes.2015;6(1):87-123.

281. American Diabetes Association, "Diagnostic Criteria for diabetes and prediabetes." DiabetesCare.2016; 37(1):515-16.

282. Adi L Tarca, Roberto Romero, Sorin Draghici, "Analysis of microarray experiments of gene expression profiling." American Journal of Obstetrics amd Gynaecology.2006;195:373-88.

283. Mandy van Hoel, Abbas Dehghan, Cornelia M., "Predicting Type 2 Diabetes Based on Polymorphisms From Geneome Wide Association Studies- A population based study."Journals ofDiabetes.2008;3(1):3122-3128.

284. Philippa J.Talmud, Jackie A Cooper, ,"Sixty five common genetics Variants

and Prediction of type 2 Diabetes."Diabetes.2015;64:1830-1840.

285. Ozsolak F, Milos PM, "RNA Sequencing: Advances, Challenges and Opprotunities." 2011;12:87-98.

286. Jenny Bryan, "Problems in gene clustering based on gene expression data.";Science direct-(2003);90:44-66.

287. Liyuan Han, Yuanyuan Li, Shwei Duan "IGF2BP2 rs11705701 polymorphisms are associated with prediabetes in a chinese population: A population based case control study.";Experimental and Therapeutics Medicine.2016;12:1849-1856.

288. Tandi E. Matsha, Carmen Phieffer, Stephen humphries, "Genome Wide DNA Methylation in mixed ancestry individuals with diabetes and prediabetes from South Africa.";International Journal of Endocrinology.2016; 3172093:1-11.

289. Talib Yusuf, Talib SH, Isolation, Qualitative and Quantitative estimation of RNA from Diabetes and Prediabetic Subjects. International Journal of Current Research.2018;10(5):69785-69787.

290. John Quackenbuck. Microarray data normalization and transformation. Nature Genetics.2002;32:496-501.

291. Donald W Pfaff, M Ian Phillips, Robert T Rubin, "Principles of Hormone/ Behavior Relations" Elsevier Inc. 2004;1(2):553149-54.

292. Robert T Rubin, Donald W Pfaff, Hormone Behavior relations of Clinical importance, Endocrine systems interacting with Brain and Behavior. Elsevier Inc.2009; 97(8):374926-40.